CW00403545

5-MINUTE

—FOR WEIGHT LOSS —

CHAIR YOGA

*Your 4-Week Journey
to Renew Your Body Image.
Low Impact Illustrated Exercises For Seniors
to Lose Belly Fat While Sitting Down,*
With Meal Plan

EVELYN TURNER

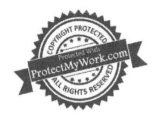

© Copyright 2023 by Evelyn Turner - All rights reserved.

This document is geared towards providing exact and reliable information in regard to the topic and issue covered. The publication is sold with the idea that the publisher is not required to render accounting, officially permitted, or otherwise, qualified services. If advice is necessary, legal or professional, a practiced individual in the profession should be ordered.

From a Declaration of Principles which was accepted and approved equally by a Committee of the American Bar Association and a Committee of Publishers and Associations. In no way is it legal to reproduce, duplicate, or transmit any part of this document in either electronic means or in printed format. Recording of this publication is strictly prohibited, and any storage of this document is not allowed unless with written permission from the publisher. All rights reserved.

The information provided herein is stated to be truthful and consistent, in that any liability, in terms of inattention or otherwise, by any usage or abuse of any policies, processes, or directions contained within is the solitary and utter responsibility of the recipient reader. Under no circumstances will any legal responsibility or blame be held against the publisher for any reparation, damages, or monetary loss due to the information herein, either directly or indirectly.

Respective authors own all copyrights not held by the publisher. The information herein is offered for informational purposes solely and is universal as such. The presentation of the information is without a contract or any type of guaranteed assurance. The trademarks that are used are without any consent, and the publication of the trademark is without permission or backing by the trademark owner. All trademarks and brands within this book are for clarifying purposes only and are owned by the owners themselves, not affiliated with this document.

Icons by Flaticon.

TABLE OF CONTENT

EXERCISES FLOWS

WARM-UP EXERCISES

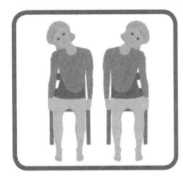

SEATED SHOULDER AND NECK ROLLS
PAG. 29

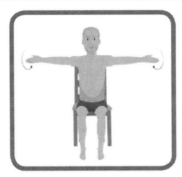

SEATED ARM CIRCLES
PAG. 30

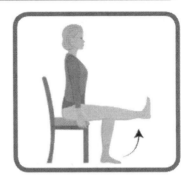

SEATED LEG LIFTS
PAG. 30

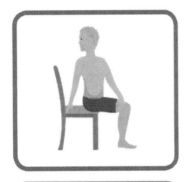

SEATED TORSO TWIST
PAG. 31

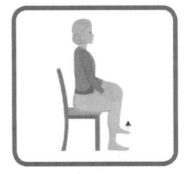

SEATED MARCHING
PAG.32

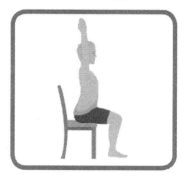

TADASANA–SEATED MOUNTAIN POSE FOR ARMS
PAG. 33

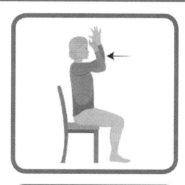

GARUDASANA ARMS–SEATED EAGLE ARMS ASANA
PAG. 33

GOMUKHASANA ARMS–SEATED COW FACE ARMS ASANA
PAG. 34

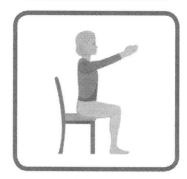

PASCHIMOTTANASANA–SEATED FORWARD BEND ASANA
PAG. 35

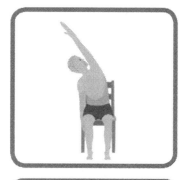

PARIVRTTA ARDHA CHANDRASANA–SEATED SIDE BEND ASANA
PAG. 36

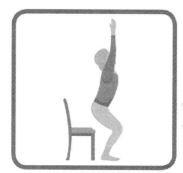

SEATED CHEST OPENING ASANA
PAG. 37

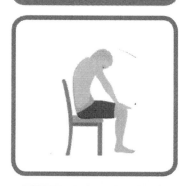

SEATED CAT-COW STRETCH
PAG. 37

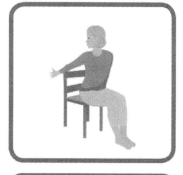

SEATED SHOULDER OPENER ASANA
PAG.38

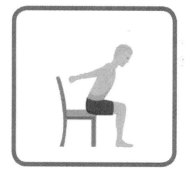

SEATED CHEST EXPANSION ASANA
PAG. 39

TARGETED ASANAS FOR SHOULDERS AND BACK

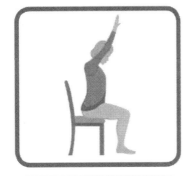

SEATED SHOULDER OPENER
WITH FORWARD FOLD
PAG. 40

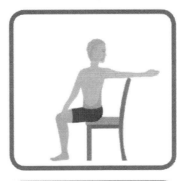

SEATED ONE ARMED
TWIST
PAG. 41

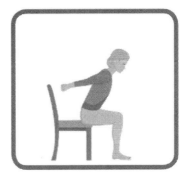

SEATED PASCHIMOTTANASANA
WITH CHEST OPENING ASANA
PAG. 42

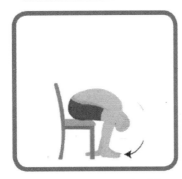

SEATED
CHILD'S POSE
PAG. 43

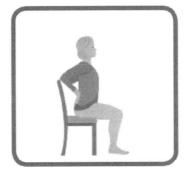

SEATED USTRANA–CAMEL
ASANA
PAG. 43

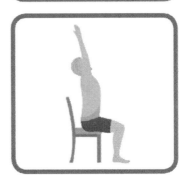

SEATED SHOULDER PRESS
ASANA
PAG. 44

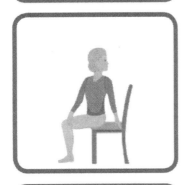

SEATED PRAYER
TWIST
PAG. 45

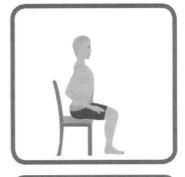

SEATED SHOULDER BLADE
SQUEEZE
PAG. 46

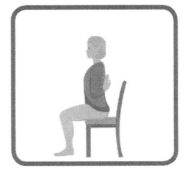

SEATED REVERSE
PRAYER POSE
PAG.46

TARGETED EXERCISES FOR CORE AND ABDOMINAL MUSCLES

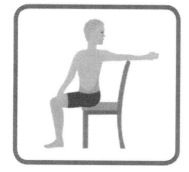

SEATED ARDHA MATSYENDRASANA–SEATED SPINAL TWIST PAG. 47

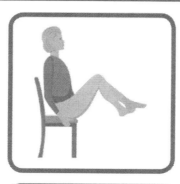

SEATED BOAT ASANA PAG. 48

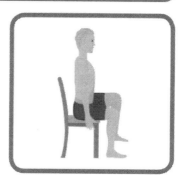

SEATED KNEE RAISE ASANA PAG. 49

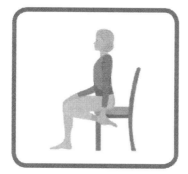

SEATED SHIN HOLD ASANA PAG. 49

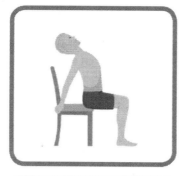

SEATED COBRA ASANA PAG. 50

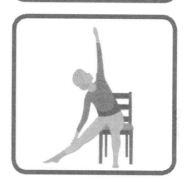

SEATED TRIANGLE ASANA PAG. 51

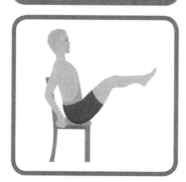

SEATED BOAT POSE WITH STRAIGHT LEGS PAG. 52

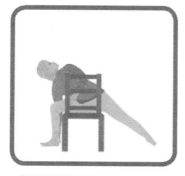

UTTHITA PARSVAKONASANA– EXTENDED SIDE ANGLE PAG.53

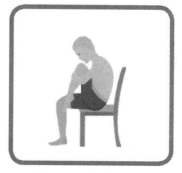

SEATED MARICHYASANA III–SIDE OBLIQUE ASANA PAG. 54

TARGETED EXERCISES FOR CORE AND ABDOMINAL MUSCLES

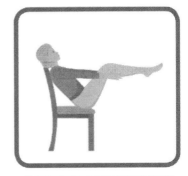

**HALF-SEATED BOAT
ASANA
PAG. 55**

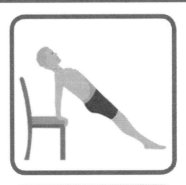

**UPWARD PLANK
POSE
PAG. 56**

TARGETED ASANAS FOR LEGS

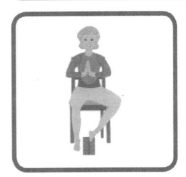

**SEATED BUTTERFLY ASANA
PAG. 57**

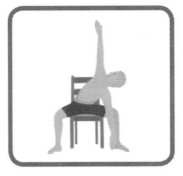

**SEATED WIDE-LEG ASANA WITH
SIDE STRETCH
PAG. 58**

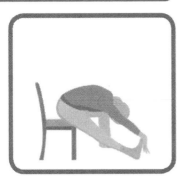

**JANU SIRSASANA–DEEP
HAMSTRING STRETCH ASANA
PAG. 59**

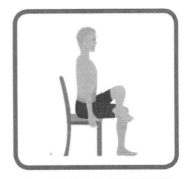

**FIGURE OF FOUR ASANA
PAG. 60**

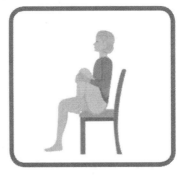

**SEATED DEEP QUAD STRETCH
PAG. 61**

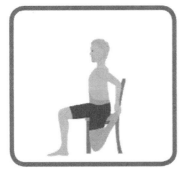

**VIRASANA HERO'S POSE–
SEATED QUAD STRETCH
PAG. 62**

TARGETED ASANAS FOR LEGS

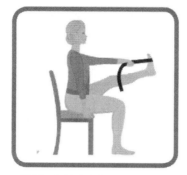

UTTHITA HASTA PADANGUSTASANA– SEATED FULL LEG STRETCH PAG. 63

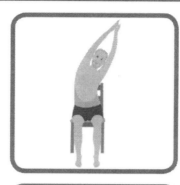

SEATED HALF-MOON WITH LEG LIFT PAG.64

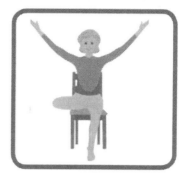

SEATED TREE ASANA PAG. 65

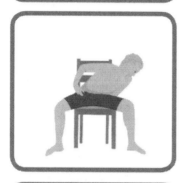

SWEEPING CIRCLES HIP OPENER PAG. 66

COOL-DOWN STRETCHES

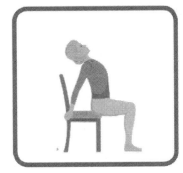

**SEATED
HEART OPENER
PAG. 67**

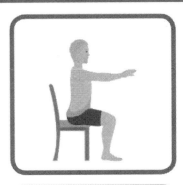

**SEATED
WRIST ROLLS
PAG. 68**

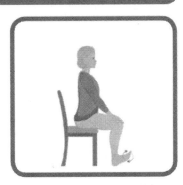

**SEATED
ANKLE CIRCLES
PAG. 68**

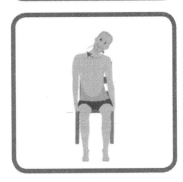

**SEATED
NECK ROLLS
PAG. 69**

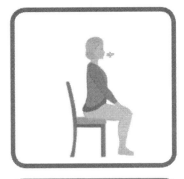

**SEATED
MEDITATION
PAG. 70**

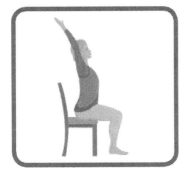

**SEATED
SUN SALUTATION
PAG. 70**

INTRODUCTION

As a child, I imagined growing older to be a world in which 50 was old and 65 was ancient—where Hollywood portrayed seniors as saucy older ladies who gathered in the kitchen to reminisce about the years gone by… "Picture this… Sicily1922," and men aged into the stereotypical grumpy or wise types, looking over neighborhood fences to bestow judgment or pearls of wisdom.

Back then, in those hay days of sitcoms featuring seniors, life was different. Comedy was satirical and as wholesome as the food we ate, and work involved a commute that required walking, regardless of the weather, and a fair amount of time standing on our feet or moving from one desk to another. It was different back then, despite the conventionalized portrayal of seniors—before the onslaught of fast-food, sedentary lifestyles, and a retirement that looked forward to seniors' homes and the occasional visit from the family we dedicated our lives to.

Modern seniors may be living longer than our predecessors but our quality of life and certainly our independence is under threat. With the slow decline of aged independence due to previous sedentary lifestyles and a lack of adequate conscious attention to movement, flexibility, and functional fitness, a group of seniors is rising up in rebellion, defiant in the face of the stereotypes they've been labeled with (Okabe et al., 2021).

Instead of sitting back and allowing the slow progress of cellular aging to overtake them, seniors are now taking a proactive approach to their health, leaving no barrier unturned in an effort to enhance their quality of life, their health, and their vitality. And yes, our bodies are not what they used to be, but that doesn't mean that accessible, gentle approaches to reclaiming our flexibility and functional fitness are not available to us.

This is the exact reason I wrote *5-Minute Chair Yoga for Weight Loss* so that everyone has the ability to improve their physical fitness, mental clarity, and flexibility without the need for rigorous postures or hip-breaking complex movements.

Throughout my 35 years working as a registered nurse, and into my retirement now as I volunteer at community centers, I've met folks like yourself who are looking to reclaim their health or who simply want to maintain an active lifestyle throughout the remainder of their lives. Three of these lovely people I've met during my career, and after, are a testament to the power of the right mindset when it's coupled with a proper health and fitness routine.

Grace, a 75-year-old retiree was diagnosed with osteoarthritis that left her with seemingly incurable pain in her joints, especially her knees and hips. With her pain not manageable, and the pain medications available to her having more risks than benefits, Grace found herself becoming increasingly less mobile. She was discouraged and felt herself slipping into depression as her once-active lifestyle seemed to be slipping from her grip. After chatting with me, a determined Grace walked into one of my chair yoga classes, and under my guidance, she began to feel the benefits of her improved strength and flexibility.

Not only did Grace improve upon her physical health but her pain and discomfort began to subside to manageable levels, making everyday tasks much easier for her to take on.

Today, Grace assists me in my classes, proving that age and pain are not insurmountable barriers and that determination with the right tools can create freedom.

It was Grace that introduced 80-year-old Robert to my class. Robert had always been an energetic, cheeky, and adventurous soul but a stroke had left him partially paralyzed on his dominant side, affecting his mobility, although not his confidence.

Robert, as upbeat as he was, longed for his independence and the unencumbered life he once had and while he knew traditional forms of yoga, didn't quite know how to use this powerful tool with his now disabled body.

With adjustment, patience, and the use of chair yoga, Robert gradually began to regain his strength and balance as his body worked to counteract the damage caused by the stroke.

Robert's goal of being able to take walks in the park unassisted once more and go to the store with limited assistance drove his determination and today, Robert embraces his disability without allowing it to reduce his quality of life or hinder his ability to live independently.

Finally, Evelyn joined my class after entering into retirement. As a school teacher, she had found her life's purpose in imparting knowledge to young minds and taking an active role in their lives. Forced into retirement, Evelyn felt that she had lost her purpose and battled with depression and anxiety that affected her sleep.

Before relenting and taking medication, Evelyn decided to try a more holistic approach to managing her anxiety and depression, and while she was skeptical, to begin with, it wasn't long before she began to feel the effects of chair yoga.

The focused breathing and mindfulness aspects of yoga taught Evelyn how to remain present in the moment, counteracting her feelings of anxiety, and this improved her overall calmness and positively affected her sleep.

With a renewed sense of belonging, Evelyn began her own community center classes, focusing on holistic treatments for depression and anxiety, teaching art therapy, and creating a new community of people who inspire her.

Chair yoga provides us with so much more than the ability to become, or remain active in our senior years—it creates a sense of independence and belonging, preserving our health and ensuring we can manage our pain, mobility, and other chronic conditions in a proactive way.

Throughout the pages of this book, you can expect to learn

- a structured 4-week program with actionable chair yoga exercises.
- easy-to-follow instructions for exercises you can do seated or with the aid of a chair that will help strengthen your muscles and improve balance.
- guided information to help you embrace a happy, healthy golden era in your life.
- meal plans so that you can nourish your body as it becomes flexible, fit, and healthy.
- practical information you can use in planning meals, working out, and continuing your journey to health long after you've turned the final pages of this book.

Now is the time to reclaim your independence, harness your inner strength, and begin a new chapter in your life using *5-Minute Yoga*—let's get started.

Chapter 1
FITNESS IN THE GOLDEN YEARS

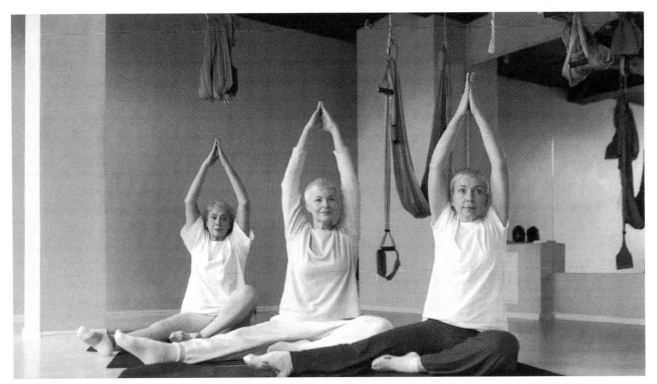

During my 6-month vacation from living, and while I was trying to reformulate what my purpose in life was after retiring from my three-plus decade nursing career I entered into a brief, yet interesting couple of months. It is now affectionately known as the "potato chip era," and looking back, it was something I probably needed to give me a not-so-gentle nudge into what I am doing with my retirement now.

At this time, and shortly before my infamous nose-dive into an overgrown mint patch in my garden, I had been mostly unaware of how my body was changing. That was until one particularly hot afternoon when I hopped in the shower to cool off and changed into my favorite summer dress… The once flowing, loose fabric now clung tightly to my belly and my arms felt uncomfortably restricted. I tugged on the dress, trying to convince myself that the fabric had shrunk in the wash or that I simply hadn't put the garment on properly.

The dress clung stubbornly to my body in places it never had and I gingerly walked over to my full-length mirror.

Like so many other women, I avoided my reflection for a large part of my life, but I hardly recognized the person staring back at me. I examined the dress first, trying to find clues as to why it was so tight, moving my gaze down from my face over my body until I fixed my eyes on my belly. "What is that?" I questioned myself as I poked the pudge that had formed around my waist. I ran through all of the reasons why my newly rounded body greeted me in the mirror.

My partner, who was also retired, hadn't developed any girth so it couldn't be our diet... I mean, I was supplying and buying the same foods and if anything, we were eating a lot better without the convenience of vending machines and a coffee shop on every corner–note, I was completely in denial about the sheer volume of snacks I was eating at this stage. "Hormones!" I declared... It had to be hormones to blame! Frustrated, I took my dress off, opting for an oversized tee and a loose pair of shorts.

Not long after, my wake-up call came and I found my way to the community center, teaching other retirees how to become fit, strong, and healthy during their golden years. The weight lingered a little while longer because once it's been accumulated it takes a while to leave when you're older, but it reaffirmed in my mind that seniors often find themselves lost when it comes to their changing bodies.

For men, hormones don't play much of a role in the later years of life. Sure... their metabolism slows to a certain extent and testosterone drops, but for the most part, eating three square meals a day while continuing to be active will have their weight remain stable.

For women, plummeting estrogen, menopause, empty nest syndrome, and falling into boredom can be our worst enemies, and if, like me, you already have a penchant for snacking, the weight can pile on, leaving us wondering where all those newly developed jiggly bits on our bodies come from.

Being fit, and maintaining a fit physique throughout our senior years is really important though, not just for our mental state of being but for our health as a whole. As we get older our bodies change and so do our nourishment needs.

Some schools of thought say that senior bodies need to revert back to toddler days when we grazed on healthy foods throughout the day, while others assert the importance of healthy fats and proteins to nourish us. Neither of these is wrong and is science-backed, along with many other recommended dietary needs and requirements, but what all this science does is confuse us and leave us wondering what we should do for our bodies.

Don't worry, I will get into this in later chapters, providing you with meal plans and shopping lists, but for now, it's important that you understand that nourishment is only one piece of the puzzle to senior health and wellness.

Why Fitness and Diet Matter in Our Senior Years

As we age, our reasons for wanting to remain fit and healthy change. Gone are the days of wanting to look great in a one-piece bathing suit or attract the ladies. We look at ourselves less in the mirror and spend more time pondering the tasks we need to get done or how we're going to keep up with our kids, grandkids, the chores around our homes, and so on... Regardless of our personal reasons for wanting to be fit and healthy, science and medicine tell us that it's absolutely vital for maintaining our independence, vitality, and quality of life.

Our physical health and mobility depend heavily on our ability to be strong and to nourish our bodies, and as we enter into our senior years, we need to shift our focus from high-intensity type training to exercise that helps improve our balance, strength, and mobility. And look, I'm not saying that cardio exercise isn't important—the ticker in our chests also needs a good workout at least once a week—but our primary focus needs to be on exercises we can do that challenge us in a holistic way. This is because as we get older joint stiffness, our range of motion, flexibility, and bone health all start to play a part in our ability to remain independent.

Once easy tasks like carrying groceries or even getting in and out of a car can become tedious or feel impossible if we don't focus on these things—strength, balance, and mobility. These forms of exercise also help us to avoid falls and fractures as well as other debilitating injuries that can threaten to throw us into depression or leave us dependent on other people.

Added to this, managing our weight while still working in harmony with our changing hormones and slowing metabolism. That doesn't mean we need to starve or deprive ourselves of the things we enjoy in life, but it does mean balancing our diet effectively with the right types of exercise and activities that are going to assist in managing our weight effectively. It also means that we need to step away from fad diets, opting for nutrient-dense foods that provide us with all of the vitamins and minerals we need to remain healthy. It's these nutrient-dense foods that will also help in keeping our hearts and minds healthy, reducing our risk of cardiovascular disease, stroke, blood pressure issues, cholesterol, and neurological diseases like Parkinson's and Alzheimer's Disease.

As we age, our bodies require an increase in certain vitamins like calcium and vitamin D to help maintain strong healthy bones. This is not only so we can avoid bone breaks but also in preventing degenerative bone diseases like osteoporosis.

Exercise, of course, also assists in building strong bones and muscles while ensuring we can keep our balance more easily.

Finally, it takes effort to concentrate on our movements, especially when we're older, and exercise can help us to remain cognitively sharp, enhancing our focus, cognitive flexibility, promoting neuroplasticity, and ensuring we get a good healthy dose of happy hormones.

Overcoming Challenges to Incorporate and Remain Consistent With Exercise and Diet

Our golden years come with a number of different challenges that we didn't have before retirement. Work and family commitments and a busy schedule that was filled with attending to the needs of others often meant we neglected ourselves—or at the very least, cited "no time" as the reason we couldn't get to the gym or be healthy and active.

But time is, for the most part, not an issue once we enter into retirement, and this means our primary go-to avoidance tactic is taken from us... and pretty swiftly at that. That's not to say other very real challenges don't crop up once we're in our golden age and it's these we will be exploring in this section.

Now, before you begin uncovering the challenges below, and the solutions of course, I'd like you to take note of your own hesitations. Most of these will be grounded in some form of fear and that's totally usual. The great thing about fear is that it can be overcome because a lot of the time, it's purely in our minds.

There is no magical switch that flipped when you turned 60 or 65, or whatever your definition of a senior is, that said you can longer do the things you used to do. You may need to adjust these things slightly while you become fitter and stronger, but your body is still capable and more than willing to be used to its fullest ability.

With that in mind, let's take a look at the challenges and obstacles you may face when incorporating exercise and a healthy diet into your life.

- You may have some physical limitations from living a sedentary life, having a chronic health condition, or an injury. Reduced muscle mass, joint stiffness, and decreased flexibility happen a lot more quickly when we are older. Add chronic health conditions and injury to the mix and you have a recipe for avoidance. There is, however, a solution, and that's to avoid high-impact activities and exercises, choosing their lower-impact counterparts—like chair yoga.
- You have a chronic health condition that limits you like heart disease, osteoporosis, or diabetes. Sure, these conditions may leave you feeling like hot, wet garbage on a sunny day most of the time but they're also a really great reason to get up, get moving, and reclaim your health. As long as you're exercising in a safe way, you're going to reap the benefits of your exercise and perhaps even reduce the symptoms of your disease. The same goes for eating healthy and studies show that a good diet that is nutrient-dense and diverse goes a long way in reducing the symptoms of certain diseases and reverses the effects of others (Willett et al., 2011).

17

- Certain medications for chronic conditions can leave you with nasty side effects including increased or decreased appetite, lowered energy levels, and even feelings of anxiety. Speak with your primary healthcare physician about alternatives to these medications and let them know that you'd like to start exercising and eating healthier so that they can prescribe the right meds for you.
- You may be experiencing some changes in your appetite as well as in your sense of taste and smell. Foods that were once appealing may now have you pushing your plate aside and that's absolutely fine. Your body is a wonderful vessel that knows what it needs and by eating healthy foods intuitively you can still nourish your body. For example, if sitting down to a full meal used to be one of the highlights of your day and now you can't stomach the thought, try serving up small "tappa-style" foods, tasting each of these mindfully before deciding what your body likes and doesn't like. If all foods are smelling and tasting awful right now, it could be an indication of a dental issue that needs to be checked out with your dentist.
- If you've experienced an injury in the past you may have issues with limited mobility or even a deep fear of injuring yourself. These fears and mobility issues are real challenges to overcome but they don't need to be the reason you don't get fit, strong, and healthy. You're going to need to tap into your inner stubbornness and tenacity to build resilience and take small steps toward reclaiming your health. It's these fears and limitations that ultimately compound our problems and by doing safe exercise you can reclaim your independence and some control over your mobility again.
- Cognitive health issues can also cause you some issues and as we become older, some things just become more and more difficult to remember. A great way to overcome this is to build a great support system by joining a community center, assigning yourself a meal and exercise buddy, or making use of technology by setting reminders for yourself.
- You may feel like you lack the knowledge to incorporate a different diet or exercise into your life now that you're in your senior years. The good news is that you're in the right place, reading the right book so that you can overcome this obstacle.
- As your time of actively working comes to an end, you may find that you have less disposable income on hand. Financial constraints are an obstacle so many seniors face and if you're one of them, this is nothing to feel ashamed of. You're doing the best you can with what you have and if no one has told you yet, I am so proud of you for taking proactive steps for your health in spite of a pretty huge challenge. This obstacle can be overcome by joining your

local community center for seniors' exercise classes, making use of coupons and feeding initiatives, and trying to form a community of seniors in a similar position as yours so that you can pool your food budgets and create bulk nutritious meals that everyone can enjoy. In joining or forming a community you're also allowing yourself to overcome the social isolation many seniors face.

- Finally, if you're still using time as a reason to avoid exercising or preparing healthy meals, then now is the time—pun intended—to find balance in your life. Keeping busy in your golden years is great but not at the expense of your health and well-being, so find the time to create a balance in your life.

Debunking Seniors Exercise and Diet Myths

Our senior years can come with some conflicting information and a lot of the time, this information has been carried down for centuries from a time before accurate science and research.

Much of this older information is based on myth and, to be honest, absolute hogwash, and in this final part of Chapter 1, we'll be debunking some of the most common of these myths.

1. **Myth**: Seniors shouldn't exercise because they could injure themselves—the reality is that proper, regular exercise is probably the most beneficial action you can take to ensure you reduce the risk of both injuries and falls.

2. **Myth**: Seniors should only focus on low-intensity exercise—while you should run off and join a high-intensity exercise class if you haven't already been attending these classes regularly, you can build yourself up to be able to enjoy all intensities and varieties of exercise. It's about being responsible with your health and your body and ensuring you're realistic about what you can do right now.

3. **Myth**: Seniors shouldn't participate in strength and weight training—fun fact… Your senior body needs strength and resistance training now more than it did when you were younger. Strength, weight, and resistance training all improve and maintain muscle mass, increase bone density, and even build muscles. Again, it's important to be realistic about what your body can do right now and build your strength up over time. Yes! That's right, you still have access to significant strength gains in your senior years if you follow a proper, regular strength training program.

4. **Myth**: It's too late to start exercising now if you've been sedentary your whole life—Absolutely not! If you're responsible and set reasonable goals for your

strength and fitness you can reap the benefits of physical activity at any stage of your life.

5. **Myth**: Seniors with chronic health conditions should avoid exercise—seniors with chronic health conditions should consult with their primary healthcare practitioner to find a set of exercises that suit their unique needs.

6. **Myth**: Seniors shouldn't do balance exercises if they're a fall risk—Balance exercise is vitally important for seniors and will help prevent falls. Balance exercises can be done in a safe environment and with assistance to ensure no falls happen.

7. **Myth**: Seniors should spend most of their time resting—rest is important but exercise is also important. Your senior years are the perfect opportunity to find proper balance in your life and take care of your needs.

8. **Myth**: Seniors shouldn't worry about their diet—nutrition becomes more important as you enter your senior years and to keep age-related diseases at bay, it's important to eat properly and regularly.

9. **Myth**: Seniors should only eat bland, easy-to-chew foods—seniors should eat a wide variety of nutritious foods and practice eating intuitively so that their bodies can be properly nourished.

10. **Myth**: Seniors need less food, regardless of how active they are—caloric needs are based on activity level and not age, and while it's true that your metabolism is slowing, this doesn't mean you need significantly less food. In fact, now is the time to nourish your body with nutrient-dense foods. Avoid calorie restrictions and opt for an increase in activity if you would like to lose weight.

11. **Myth**: Seniors need to take nutritional supplements to meet their nutritional needs—the nutraceutical industry is almost wholly unregulated and mostly a money-making scheme that taps into the fears of people. If you're eating a wide variety of foods that are nutritious and natural, and you haven't specifically been prescribed a supplement by your doctor, there's no need to supplement with pills and shakes.

12. **Myth:** Seniors can't lose weight for their health—You can gain and lose weight at any stage of your life for your health. What you shouldn't be doing is following restrictive fad diets that could damage your health. Instead, opt for nutritious healthy foods that are good for your body and increase activity levels so that you can create a calorie deficit.

13. **Myth**: Seniors shouldn't eat fats—healthy fats should be consumed at every stage of your life while minimizing the intake of unhealthy fats. That means eating nuts, avocados, whole eggs, dairy, fatty fish, and even dark chocolate.

14. **Myth**: Seniors should reduce their water intake—while you may not feel as thirsty as you used to, it's really important that you continue to drink water throughout the course of the day. The WHO recommends up to 12 ounces of water every day that can be sipped slowly.

15. **Myth**: Seniors shouldn't eat carbohydrates—your body needs carbohydrates! In fact, carbohydrates should be the primary source of your energy intake throughout the day. For seniors, healthy carbohydrates should make up between 45 and 65% of your diet. Healthy carbs, fruits, and vegetables include bananas, blueberries, sweet potatoes, chickpeas, and corn. Whole grains including oats, quinoa, and buckwheat are also great sources of healthy carbohydrates.

Our golden years are not that different from the years preceding them and while our bodies may not feel the same, or may require us to make some adjustments to the way we get our exercise or nutrition, our health should remain our number one priority.

While some of us may have challenges we need to overcome, like mobility, illness, or injury issues, we can still enjoy a full life that embraces health and fitness.

Modified exercises like chair yoga provide us with the unique opportunity to empower our bodies and our minds as we age, becoming strong, fit, and capable and securing our independence well into our retirement year.

Chapter 2

THE SCIENCE AND BENEFITS OF CHAIR YOGA

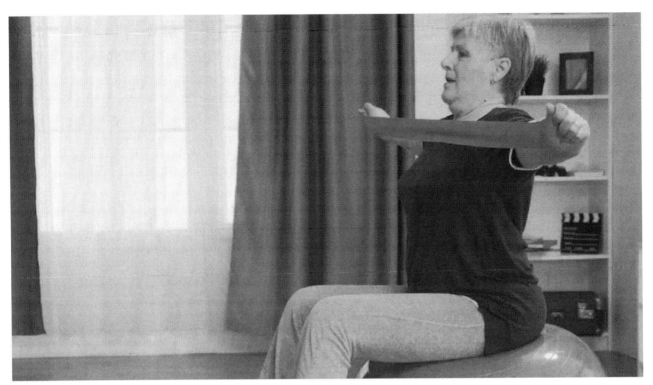

The golden years don't need to be ones in which we slowly watch and feel our bodies slow down and our strength fade. In fact, keeping up with a great diet and sufficient exercise is really important as we enter retirement but often our fear of falling, age-related disease, and joint stiffness can present us with what feels like an insurmountable roadblock.

What we need to be able to do is create a sustainable routine in which we can exercise safely while still enjoying the powerful benefits of exercise.

Chair yoga is one of these gentle, but formidable exercises that offer us the opportunity to not only cultivate a mind-body connection but also ensure we are able to safely and confidently improve our strength and flexibility, and control our weight while we build strong, healthy muscles.

As the name suggests, chair yoga is an adaptation of traditional yoga that has been specially formulated for people who have balance and mobility issues, or other physical limitations. It provides people like you and me with the opportunity to reap the benefits of traditional yoga without the need for complex postures, or near-perfect balance.

The exact history of chair yoga is unknown, but many credit this adapted form of yoga to the now legendary guru, Bellur Krishnamachar Sundararaja Iyengar–BKS Iyengar.

Born in 1918 in a ruler village in India, Iyengar would become one of the most influential and significant figures in the world of yoga and a catalyst for the international popularity of yoga around the globe. But Iyengar's life wasn't an easy one and he suffered from a multitude of health issues including typhoid, malaria, and tuberculosis.

At age 16, the young Iyengar would join his guru brother-in-law to study yoga and while he initially faced challenges because of his weak, frail body, through determination and dedication, Iyengar would transform his body and life.

Iyengar's yoga style would later be known as "Iyengar Yoga," a style of the practice that focused on precision and alignment while using props to help perform the numerous yoga postures–asanas.

This methodical approach to finding balance and harmony within the body and mind gained popularity among people who were previously unable to reap the benefits of yoga and won numerous awards and recognition around the world.

Iyengar passed away at the age of 95 but his legacy continues through the variations of his practice.

The Benefits of Chair Yoga

Chair yoga's primary benefit lies in its accessibility and it opens the doors to the benefits of traditional yoga without excluding those who have mobility or other health issues. For seniors in particular, chair yoga is a way to rejuvenate bodies and minds and find solace in the gentle stretches as well as the calming breathwork that are a hallmark of yoga, all while having the security of a chair.

Chair yoga empowers older adults to be able to maintain their independence while improving their flexibility and enhancing their physical and mental health.

But chair yoga isn't only for seniors and a new wave of office workers has embraced chair yoga as a way to combat desk-bound hours, combating the symptoms of a forced sedentary life. For those with disabilities and other physical limitations, chair yoga helps them to embrace their bodies' unique capabilities while becoming stronger and fitter as they improve upon their ability to use their bodies to their fullest abilities.

Aside from this primary benefit, chair yoga has been shown to

- improve flexibility through the institution of gentle stretches that help improve muscle function. This, in turn, makes daily movements much easier and reduces the risk of falls and injuries.
- effectively enhance muscle strength, particularly in the lower body, back, and core muscles, improving posture and ensuring physical stability is enhanced.
- improve joint mobility and reduce stiffness and discomfort in the body. Proponents of chair yoga report relief in their shoulders, knees, and hips within a few short weeks of practicing chair yoga.
- improve balance and stability which helps to reduce the risk of falls, especially in seniors and for those with disabilities.
- reduce stress with the use of mindful breathing and stretches, reducing cortisol levels in the body and helping the body heal.
- improve circulation within the body and improve heart and lung health.
- enhance body awareness through mindful movements and being aware of the physical sensations within the body.
- alleviate the chronic pain that is associated with conditions like arthritis and fibromyalgia. Chair yoga is also known to relieve back and joint pain.
- improve mental focus and mindfulness enhancing cognitive function, clarity, and focus.
- assist in creating a low-impact workout that doesn't create stress on joints and muscles. This means exercise can be done even when recovering from injuries and surgery.
- increase energy levels and reduce fatigue so that energy levels can be sustained throughout the course of the day.
- improve emotional well-being by incorporating mindfulness and meditation into an exercise routine. This helps to reduce anxiety and depression and instill a sense of optimism for life.
- reduce muscle tension by not only promoting relaxation but also increasing overall muscle strength.
- improve breathing by increasing lung capacity, respiratory function, and oxygen intake. The breathwork involved in yoga also increases breath awareness, preventing the onset of panic attacks or other anxiety-related issues.

Chair yoga may not be the cure-all for the issues we face as we age but it does offer a number of benefits to help improve our quality of life as well as our mental and physical well-being.

The independence we build as we become stronger and more capable helps to remind us that our lives are by no means over and that we are merely entering into a new chapter of living where we get to enjoy the fruits of our labors.

Chair Yoga for Weight Loss and Improved Physique

Before getting into how chair yoga can contribute to weight loss and improved physique, it's important that we explore how our bodies use fuel—the food we eat—and how weight gain happens.

Everything we eat and drink, except water, contains calories. While most of us think that calories are these scary things we need to count or that contribute toward fat and increasing weight, they're actually just a unit of measurement of energy and are no different from volts and watts.

Our bodies need a specific number of calories every day to fuel the processes that keep us alive. This includes breathing, our heart beating, sleeping, thinking, metabolism, immune system, and so on. This basic calorie number is called our resting metabolic rate and it assumes we are doing nothing extra to burn fuel in our bodies. Increased activity in the form of walking, brushing our teeth, getting dressed, going to the store, and other daily tasks require additional energy that needs to be converted from the food we eat or from energy reserves in our body in the form of fat or glucose.

One of the biggest myths seniors are subjected to is that their bodies don't need as many calories as younger bodies and while this is somewhat true, the difference in caloric intake is miniscule.

The average adult male requires between 2,400 and 2,600 calories every day to fuel and sustain their body; the average adult female needs between 1,800 and 2,200 calories. Now, as we enter into our senior years we're told that our metabolism slows but this slowing is based solely on two factors—a reduction in lean muscle mass and an increase in sedentary habits. If we were to assume this is correct, the average senior male would require 2,000 to 2,400 calories every day and the average senior female would need 1,600 to 2,000 calories—so a 200-calorie difference between seniors and middle-aged adults. To put this into perspective, four strips of bacon, three boiled medium-sized eggs, two tablespoons of peanut butter, and one 8-ounce glass of milk all contain 200 calories.

The issue with believing this myth about reduced calories is that we're inadvertently causing harm to our bodies by not providing enough fuel and we're creating a situation in which we're actually perpetuating the myth. The reason for this is muscle requires more fuel in the form of calories. The more muscle mass we have, the more calories we need to take in to fuel them. Without the right number of calories being consumed, our bodies begin to waste, beginning with our muscles. Fewer calories and exercise equals less muscle mass creating a reduction in lean muscle and weakness that leads to a sedentary lifestyle… and we create the myth.

Right, now that we understand what calories are, let's look at weight gain and loss. When we eat more calories than our bodies need, our bodies store this energy as fat. Over time, this fat can compound and create visceral fat which is a hard form of these fatty substances that settle around our organs. Visceral fat is really, really bad for our health and can cause a plethora of issues for us including heart and cardiovascular, as well as liver disease.

The other form of fat that accumulates in our bodies is called subcutaneous fat and this is the jiggly stuff we see on our bellies, arms, around our hips, and on our thighs. Subcutaneous fat is more easy to lose than visceral fat but all fat is lost by burning these energy reserves and creating a calorie deficit.

I'd like to get some things squared away when it comes to calorie deficits before we continue on in this chapter.

A calorie deficit is *not* starving ourselves or drastically reducing the number of calories eaten in a day. In fact, cutting just 200 calories from our current diet adds up to 1,400 calories every week and around 6,000 calories in a calendar month. This is more than sufficient to lose around one pound of fat per month—which is healthy weight loss, by the way. Next, we don't actually need to reduce our food intake for us to put our bodies into a calorie deficit.

Exercise is activity and activity burns more calories in our bodies. If we were to continue eating exactly the way we do now but increased our activity levels, we'd burn more calories. Finally, the number on the scale means absolutely nothing! The reason for this is that muscle is more dense than fat. Technically speaking, we could lose pounds of fat while increasing our muscle mass and our weight would increase… *but*, we would be more healthy!

What we need to focus on, especially as we age is not how much we weigh but how strong, fit, and mobile we feel.

Debunking the High-Intensity Myth

We live in a world of instant gratification and disposable, well, just about everything. In this new world, where everything is designed to "improve" our way of life—and I use that phrase very loosely—the health and fitness industry emerged.

New exercise trends that promise to burn hundreds of calories in a few short minutes and target every muscle group have become all the rage and proponents of these exercises state that the only way to effectively lose weight and keep it off is to practice high-intensity forms of exercise.

To better understand why these statements simply aren't true, we need to break down how high-intensity and low-intensity exercise works on our bodies.

High-intensity workouts, like spinning classes, cross-fit, and high-intensity interval training (HIIT) are designed to ramp up our heart rates and activate our fast twitch muscles which help us move quickly in short, sharp bursts.

Now, while I am not denying that high-intensity workouts do burn a whole lot of calories, they're designed for, and shouldn't be practiced, for more than 30 minutes—don't let adverts for 60-minute classes fool you… a substantial amount of this time is used for warming-up and cooling-down periods. During these 30-minute exercise periods, high-intensity workouts burn around 500 calories, give or take depending on weight, stature, and fitness levels.

These workouts push us into our anaerobic or VO2 max thresholds and according to "fitness experts" this is where we want to be… *if* we're peak-performing athletes, which we're not, of course. So, 500 calories burned for 30 minutes of pain.

Low and mid-intensity workouts, like chair yoga, aqua aerobics, and wall pilates, also increase our heart rate but instead of being in the VO2 max or anaerobic thresholds, our heart rate remains in the aerobic or intensive thresholds. When we are in these areas of our heart rate we can sustain our exercise for longer periods of time, achieving up to an hour of exercise at a time.

These types of exercises engage our slow-twitch muscle fibers that are used to fuel and build our muscles and create endurance and fitness. Low and mid-intensity exercise burns fewer calories in the first 30 minutes of exercising but more calories in the second half of the workout. These kinds of exercise burn between 500 and 1,000 calories per hour which technically means we burn exactly the same amount of calories without the risk of injury or the pain and discomfort associated with high-intensity workouts.

The reason low and medium-intensity exercises are so effective in burning calories is because they increase muscle mass, burn off fat more effectively, and improve our endurance. What we need to understand as seniors is that less is more when it comes to the impact and intensity of our exercise routine. Gentle, low-impact exercise with a healthy, balanced diet is far more constructive than joining a spinning class and hoping our joints won't suffer for it.

Now that we understand how calories work, and the difference between the types of exercise, it's time to get into our workout.

Chapter 3
ILLUSTRATED CHAIR YOGA EXERCISES
FOR WEIGHT LOSS

We now have all the information we need to embark on our journey to mobility, a stronger body, and renewed independence. This chapter will break down each of our targeted muscle groups. These exercises include a warm-up as well as a cool-down section. It is incredibly important that we take the time to warm up and cool down so that we can prevent this risk of injuries like muscle strains as well as helping to combat post-exercise stiffness.

These exercises are designed so that you need no equipment other than a sturdy chair and clear workout space.

Before instituting any new workout routine, it's a good idea to consult with your doctor to discuss any physical or disease-related limitations you may have. Always be sensible with what your current capabilities are, and work diligently at perfecting your poses rather than trying to push your body which could cause an injury.

Remember, chair yoga is a gentle, yet effective form of exercise, breathe deeply into your poses, focus on form, and celebrate as your body changes and becomes stronger and more flexible.

Warm-Up Exercises

Warming up before we exercise is absolutely critical to help us prevent muscle strains and injury. The primary reason we warm up is to gradually raise our body's core temperature so that our cardiovascular system, muscles, and mind all prepare for the exercise we're about to do.

When we warm up we gradually increase the blood flow to our muscles, enhance oxygen and nutrients to our organs and muscles and improve our lubrication in our joints. It's important that we take the time to warm up our entire body, even if we're only going to work out one particular group of muscles for the day.

As with the other exercises contained in this book, each of these warm-up movements can be done while you're seated in a comfortable chair.

Make sure to perform each of these warm-up exercises in a controlled way and don't rush.

Breathe deeply throughout these movements to help increase the oxygen flow in your muscles.

Remember to listen to your body and modify the movements according to your own unique needs and comfort levels.

With persistence and time, you will be able to complete these movements without modification as your body becomes stronger.

SEATED SHOULDER AND NECK ROLLS | *DIFFICULTY–EASY*

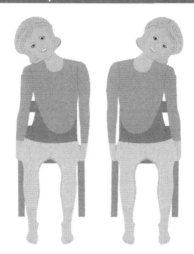

- Take a seat in your chair.
- Sit tall and make sure your feet are flat on the ground.
- Place your hands, palm down on your thighs.
- Inhale deeply and lift your shoulders up towards your ears.
- Begin to exhale slowly as you roll your shoulders back and towards your spine.
- Return your shoulders to a neutral position.
- Bring your focus to your head.
- Look up towards the ceiling and inhale deeply.
- Slowly roll your head around, exhaling as you roll.
- Once your head has reached its starting position of staring at the ceiling, return it to a neutral position.
- Return your focus to your shoulders.
- Alternate between these two movements, shoulders and neck for 10 repetitions, making sure to focus on your breath and being mindful of how your muscles are loosening.

SEATED ARM CIRCLES | *DIFFICULTY–EASY*

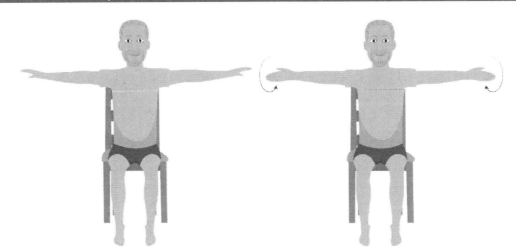

- Remain seated, sitting tall with your feet flat on the floor.
- Slowly lift your arms, extending them out to your sides at shoulder height. Try to keep your arms as straight as possible.
- Inhale deeply and begin to make small circular movements with your arms.
- Try to complete five forward movements and five backward movements.
- Total repetitions should be 10.

SEATED LEG LIFTS | *DIFFICULTY–EASY TO MEDIUM*

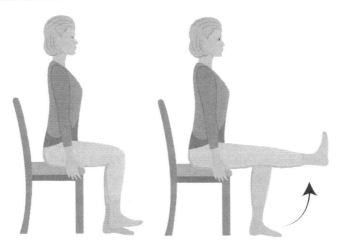

- Shift your body toward the edge of the chair but not too close to the edge. You should still feel balanced when sitting tall.
- Place your hands on the sides of the chair.
- Inhale deeply, and focus your attention on your right leg.
- Exhale and lift your right leg off the floor, aiming to extend it out straight in front of you.
- Hold this position for a count of three and lower your leg back down in a controlled manner.
- Now, inhale deeply again, changing your focus to your left leg.

- Exhale and lift your left leg off the floor, aiming to extend it out straight in front of you.
- Hold this position for a count of three and lower your leg back down in a controlled manner.
- Alternate your legs and aim for 10 repetitions on each leg. If you cannot do 10 full repetitions just yet, don't worry about it, you'll get there soon.

SEATED TORSO TWIST | *DIFFICULTY–EASY TO MEDIUM*

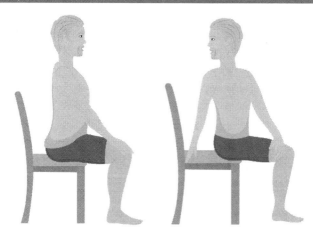

- Sit back in your chair once more.
- Return your legs to a neutral position, feet on the floor.
- Place your hands, palm down, on your thighs.
- Sit up tall and straight and inhale deeply as you stretch your spine upward.
- As you exhale, gently twist your torso, from the hips upward, to your right side–try to look over your shoulder.
- Hold this position for a count of five before returning to a neutral position.
- Inhale deeply again, stretching your spine upward.
- As you exhale, gently twist your torso, from the hips upward, to your left side– try to look over your shoulder.
- Hold this position for a count of five before returning to a neutral position.
- Repeat this exercise, making sure to focus on your breath and form for 10 repetitions.
- Make sure not to push yourself too hard when twisting your spine. The point is to comfortably stretch your back, not hurt yourself.

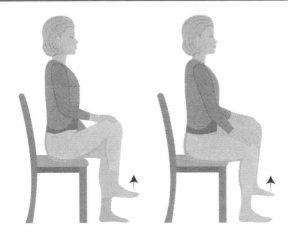

- Remain in your current seated position with a straight spine and feet flat on the floor.
- Inhale deeply.
- As you begin to exhale, lift your right knee up towards your chest–you may place your hands on the side of your chair if you feel unbalanced or directly in front of you for a more advanced warm-up.
- Immediately return your right knee to its starting position.
- Lift your left knee towards your chest and immediately return it to its starting position.
- Your exercise should look like you're marching on the spot.
- Repeat this exercise for a count of 30– or 15 repetitions on each leg.

Each of these exercises is designed to warm up your whole body. If you are following our workout plan, I would recommend that you spend just a little extra time on whichever targeted exercise you're doing on a day. Remember, the point is to build up your strength gradually. If you cannot get through these repetitions it is nothing to be embarrassed of–you'll become strong and fit in no time.

Targeted Asanas for Arms and Chest

Chair yoga, as you know, comes with a whole lot of different benefits that help to improve our strength and flexibility. Once your body is warmed up you can choose to focus on specific targeted areas of your body that you feel may be weak, or opt for a full-body seated yoga session. If you're not too sure what workouts to do on what days, feel free to make use of our workout guide in Chapter 4.

Each of these asanas, or poses, should be completed mindfully, paying attention to your breath and to how your body feels when doing them. Feel free to modify these asanas to suit your specific limitations or comfort levels until you are able to complete them without pain.

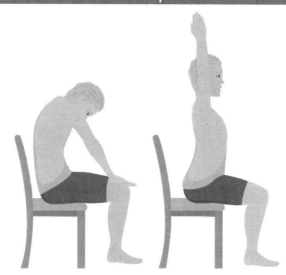

- Sit comfortably on your chair, spine tall and stretched and feet flat on the floor, hip-width apart.
- Place your hands on your thighs, palms facing down and inhale deeply.
- As you begin to exhale, raise your arms towards the ceiling. Try to keep your arms as straight as possible without lifting or tensing your shoulders.
- With your arms up, reaching for the ceiling, focus your attention on your breath.
- Inhale deeply through your nose, hold your breath for a count of three, and exhale through your mouth.
- Aim to hold your pose for three full repetitions of your breath at first, working your way up to ten repetitions of your breath.
- Make sure to hold focus on your breath and your form throughout the asana.

GARUDASANA ARMS—SEATED EAGLE ARMS ASANA | *DIFFICULTY—MEDIUM*

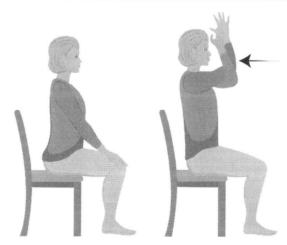

- Remain in your seated position, feet flat on the floor, and spine straight.
- Place your hand on your thighs, palms facing down.

33

- Inhale deeply, lifting and extending both arms in front of you until they're at shoulder height.
- As you begin to exhale, cross your right arm over your left arm until your right elbow rests on your left arm above the elbow.
- Try to touch the palm of your right hand to the top of your left hand without your elbows losing contact—if this pose is too easy for you, you can try intertwining your forearms until the palms of your hands touch.
- Inhale deeply through your nose, hold your breath for a count of three, and exhale through your mouth while maintaining this position.
- Now, repeat this pose on the other side, crossing your left arm over the right.
- Aim to hold your pose on each side for three full repetitions of your breath at first, working your way up to ten repetitions of your breath.
- Return your arms to their resting position.

GOMUKHASANA ARMS–SEATED COW FACE ARMS ASANA | *DIFFICULTY–MEDIUM TO HARD*

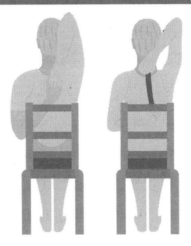

- Remain in your seated position, feet flat on the floor, and spine straight and tall.
- Inhale deeply.
- As you begin to exhale, slowly extend your right arm up toward the ceiling.
- Make sure to keep your shoulders in a neutral position throughout this movement.
- Once your arm is fully extended above your head, bend your right elbow and reach your hand down towards your spine in the center of your shoulder blades.
- Now, extend your left arm out to the side of your body until it is at shoulder height.
- Bend your left elbow and try to reach for your right hand.

- If your hands don't touch, that's absolutely fine, try using a strap or a towel that you can drape from your top hand to the bottom one so that you can remain in this position for the required number of breaths.
- Inhale deeply through your nose, hold your breath for a count of three, and exhale through your mouth while maintaining this position.
- Now, repeat this pose on the other side, with your right hand reaching for the left.
- Aim to hold your pose on each side for three full repetitions of your breath at first, working your way up to five repetitions of your breath.
- Return your arms to their resting position.

PASCHIMOTTANASANA–SEATED FORWARD BEND ASANA | *DIFFICULTY–EASY*

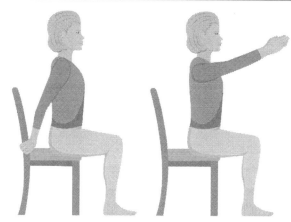

- Remain in your seated position, feet flat on the floor, and spine straight and tall.
- Extend your arms slowly behind you, palms facing down and fingers toward your body.
- Inhale deeply as you lengthen your spine and try to extend your arms further back.
- Bring your focus to your breath.
- As you exhale, try to interlock your fingers so that you're holding your own hands—if this exercise is too easy for you, interlock your hands and try lifting your arms up toward your shoulders slightly.
- Aim to hold your pose on each side for three full repetitions of your breath at first, working your way up to eight repetitions of your breath.
- Return your arms to their resting position.

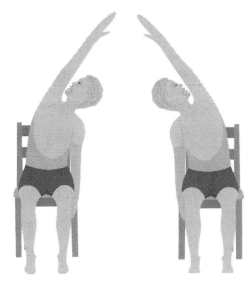

- Remain in your seated position, feet flat on the floor, and spine straight and tall.
- Inhale deeply and slowly reach your right arm up toward the ceiling. Try to keep your hand neutral and relaxed and your elbow very slightly bent.
- As you begin to exhale, gently lean your body to the left without lifting your rear off your seat.
- Bend over as far as you comfortably can–you can rest your left hand on the chair if you're feeling unbalanced.
- Bring your focus to your breath and hold the asana for a count of five breaths.
- Return to your neutral position.
- Inhale deeply and slowly reach your left arm up toward the ceiling. Try to keep your hand neutral and relaxed and your elbow very slightly bent.
- As you begin to exhale, gently lean your body to the right without lifting your rear off your seat.
- Bend over as far as you comfortably can–you can rest your right hand on the chair if you're feeling unbalanced.
- Bring your focus to your breath and hold the asana for a count of five breaths.
- Return to your neutral position.

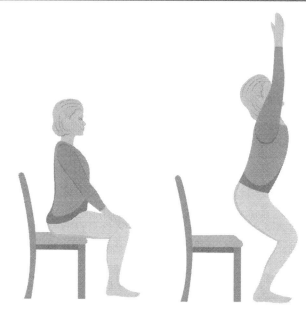

- Remain in your seated position, feet flat on the floor, and spine straight and tall.
- Inhale deeply and lift your hands to chest height.
- Bend your elbows and bring the palms of your hands together, interlacing your fingers.
- Exhale and bring focus to your breath.
- Begin to lift your arms up towards the ceiling. Do not release your hands.
- Now, slowly push backward, opening up your chest and encouraging your shoulder blades to touch.
- Bring your focus to your breath and hold the asana for a count of five breaths.
- Return to your neutral position.

SEATED CAT-COW STRETCH | *DIFFICULTY–MEDIUM*

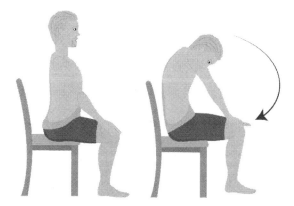

- Remain in your seated position, feet flat on the floor, and spine straight and tall.
- Place your hands on your knees, palms down.

- Inhale deeply and with your inhale arch your back, lifting your chest forward.
- Slowly lift your head towards the ceiling—Cow pose.
- As you begin to exhale, round your back, bringing your head down towards your chest. Concentrate on keeping your back rounding on your exhale movement—Cat pose.
- Inhale again, arching your back, lifting your chest forward, and bringing your gaze towards the ceiling.
- Repeat your exhale movement.
- Move between the cow and cat pose for a total of five breaths.

SEATED SHOULDER OPENER ASANA | *DIFFICULTY—EASY*

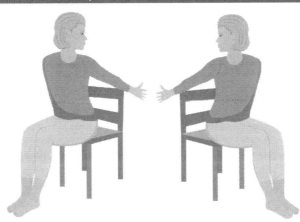

- Remain in your seated position, feet flat on the floor, and spine straight and tall.
- Inhale and begin to lift your right arm straight out in front of you until it is at shoulder height.
- Exhale and turn your palm outward, towards the wall.
- Bring focus to your breath and slowly sweep your right arm out to the side.
- Reach as far back as you possibly can without placing strain on your muscles or bending your arm.
- Hold this position for three breath counts.
- Return your right arm to a neutral position, palm down on your thigh.
- Inhale and begin to lift your left arm straight out in front of you until it is at shoulder height.
- Exhale and turn your palm outward, towards the wall.
- Bring focus to your breath and slowly sweep your left arm out to the side.
- Reach as far back as you possibly can without placing strain on your muscles or bending your arm.
- Hold this position for three breath counts.
- Return to a neutral position.

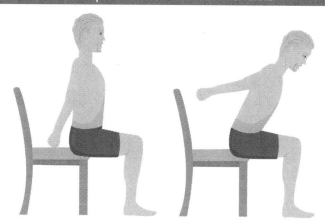

- Remain in your seated position, feet flat on the floor, and spine straight and tall.
- Shift forward slightly on your chair, creating some space between your back and the back support.
- Inhale deeply and begin to move your hands toward your lower back–arms can be bent or straight, it depends on the space available to you.
- Clasp your hands together, palms touching, and exhale–if you cannot clasp your hands behind your back, feel free to use a towel or strap to connect your hands.
- Bring focus to your breath and begin to lift your arms slightly up your spine. Make sure your shoulders remain relaxed and in a neutral position.
- If you are not feeling the stretch in your chest, try opening your chest more by bringing your shoulder blades together.
- Hold this position for five breath counts.
- Return to a neutral position.

Once you have finished working out a specific area of your body it is a good idea to remain seated in your neutral position for a few breath counts. Get up slowly from your work out and if you feel dizzy, remain seated until the feeling passes.

Targeted Asanas for Shoulders and Back

Each of these asanas in this section is designed to help target your shoulder and back muscles. It's critical that you remain mindful and aware during these poses so that you don't place strain on your muscles. Your shoulders and back are really important for completing everyday tasks.

Everything from lifting and carrying to reaching overhead and retrieving things involves these muscles.

While these muscles are not usually used in isolation and require a strong core, legs, or chest to help in these tasks, it's still vitally important that we ensure they're strong so that we can maintain a balance and equilibrium between the work our muscles need to do when we are active. Feel free to modify these asanas to suit your specific limitations or comfort levels until you are able to complete them without pain.

SEATED SHOULDER OPENER WITH FORWARD FOLD | *DIFFICULTY–EASY*

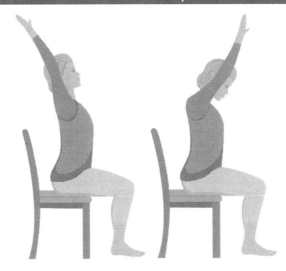

- Sit comfortably on your chair, spine tall and stretched and feet flat on the floor, hip-width apart–this is your neutral position.
- Place your hands on your knees, palms down.
- Inhale deeply.
- As you begin to exhale, slowly lift your hands up toward the ceiling until they're above your head.
- Clasp your hands above your head in a modified prayer position and reach up toward the ceiling as high as you can.
- Bring focus to your breath and hold for two full breath counts.
- Now, without loosening your hands or bending your arms, slowly bend forward from your hips-keep your spine straight and your shoulders relaxed and in a neutral position.
- Once you reach a comfortable position with your toro, bring focus back to your breath.
- Hold this asana for a total of five breath counts.
- Return to your neutral position.

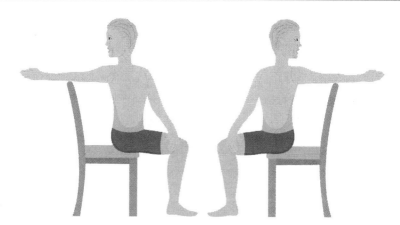

- Remain in your seated position, feet flat on the floor, and spine straight and tall.
- Inhale deeply, lengthening your spine upward towards the ceiling and your chest outward.
- As you begin to exhale, lift your right arm out and toward your side—don't bend your elbow, if possible.
- Bring focus to your breath, and inhale slowly as you sweep your right arm across your chest, trying to lie your bicep horizontally across your chest—if you cannot place your bicep on your chest, hold your arm in the most comfortable, straight position.
- Hold this position for a total of five breath counts.
- Return to your neutral position.
- Now, inhale deeply, lengthening your spine upward towards the ceiling and your chest outward.
- As you begin to exhale, lift your left arm out and toward your side—don't bend your elbow, if possible.
- Bring focus to your breath, and inhale slowly as you sweep your left arm across your chest, trying to lie your bicep horizontally across your chest—if you cannot place your bicep on your chest, hold your arm in the most comfortable, straight position.
- Hold this position for a total of five breath counts.
- Should you not be able to comfortably hold your arm in its position straight across your chest, feel free to bend your elbow slightly and clasp the opposite arm's bicep while you hold your asana for the required breath counts.
- Return to a neutral position.

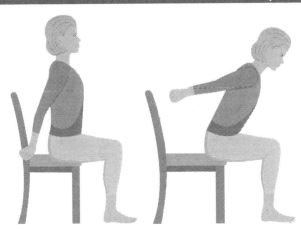

- Remain in your seated position, feet flat on the floor, and spine straight and tall.
- Extend your arms slowly behind you, palms facing down and fingers toward your body.
- Inhale deeply as you lengthen your spine and try to extend your arms further back.
- Bring your focus to your breath.
- As you exhale, try to interlock your fingers so that you're holding your own hands—if this exercise is too easy for you, interlock your hands and try lifting your arms up toward your shoulders slightly.
- Now, open your chest, bringing your shoulder blades as close together as you can.
- Lift your head slightly toward the ceiling, allowing air to fill your lungs with each inhale
- Aim to hold your pose on each side for three full repetitions of your breath at first, working your way up to five repetitions of your breath.
- This asana can be quite difficult to begin with. If you find you are struggling, make sure to place focus on what you can do, choosing to place focus on technique rather than trying to get into the asana perfectly.
- Return your arms, chest, and shoulders to their resting position.

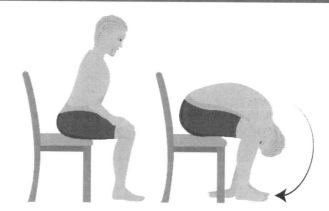

- Shift your rear towards the front of your chair.
- Make sure your feet are flat on the floor and about hip-width apart.
- Test your balance by leaning forward slightly and adjust your position if necessary.
- Inhale deeply and draw focus to your breath.
- As you exhale, slowly bend forward from your hips. Keep your spine straight as you bend forward.
- Drop your arms down and position them so that they're grasping the bottom of your chair legs. If you cannot reach the chair legs, grasp the part of your own legs that is comfortable for you.
- Aim to hold your pose for five full repetitions of your breath at first, working your way up to eight repetitions of your breath.
- Slowly return to your starting position, concentrating on your breath and your balance.
- Only move on to your next asana once you have reorientated yourself.

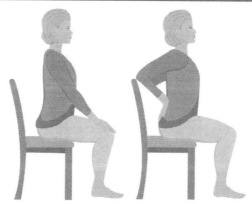

- Remain in your seated position, feet flat on the floor, and spine straight and tall.
- Move forward in your chair slightly so that there is enough space between your back and your chair to place your hands on your lower back.

43

- Shift your feet slightly so that they're slightly less than shoulder-width apart.
- Inhale slowly and begin to move your hands towards your lower back. Keep your fingers pointing down and get comfortable—you can clasp your hands together if you're able to, or rest them on your back if you cannot. Make sure your fingers continue to point downwards towards the floor.
- Exhale and bring focus to your breath.
- On your next inhale, gently open and lift your chest, and arch your lower back forwards, away from the backrest.
- Exhale slowly.
- Aim to hold your pose for five full repetitions of your breath at first, working your way up to eight repetitions of your breath.
- If you find this asana to be too easy, try clasping your hands around the backrest of your chair and lifting your head towards the ceiling.
- Return to your neutral position.

SEATED SHOULDER PRESS ASANA | *DIFFICULTY—EASY TO HARD (MODIFICATION DEPENDENT)*

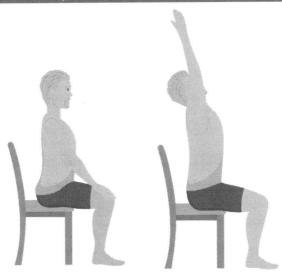

If you like, you can hold a small ball or bottle of water in each hand for this exercise to add more resistance and build more strength. Otherwise, use your own body weight, and as your strength gradually increases you can begin to add weight.

- Remain in your seated position, feet flat on the floor, and spine straight and tall.
- Place your hands on your thighs, palms facing up towards the ceiling.
- Inhale gently and bring focus to your breath.
- As you begin to exhale, slowly lift your arms up towards the ceiling until they are fully extended.
- Hold your arms above your head for three full breath counts before returning them to your thighs.

- Complete five repetitions of this pose, working your way up to 10 repetitions. Once you can easily do 10 repetitions, increase the weight you are holding.
- Return to your neutral position.

SEATED PRAYER TWIST | *DIFFICULTY–EASY*

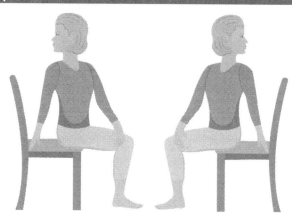

- Remain in your seated position, feet flat on the floor, and spine straight and tall.
- Inhale deeply and place your right hand on your left knee.
- Exhale and place your left hand on your chair.
- Inhale once more, lengthening your spine upwards toward the ceiling.
- As you begin to exhale, gently twist your torso toward your left side—try to look over your left shoulder.
- Hold this position for five full breath counts.
- Return to your neutral position.
- Now, inhale deeply and place your left hand on your right knee.
- Exhale and place your right hand on your chair.
- Inhale once more, lengthening your spine upwards toward the ceiling.
- As you begin to exhale, gently twist your torso toward your right side—try to look over your right shoulder.
- Hold this position for three full breath counts.
- Return to your neutral position.

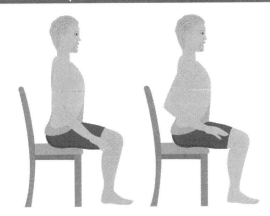

- Remain in your seated position, feet flat on the floor, and spine straight and tall.
- Place your hands on your thighs, palms facing down.
- Inhale deeply and open your chest, squeezing your shoulder blades together.
- Hold for two full breath counts.
- Release your position and remain in the neutral seated position for two full breath counts.
- Repeat this movement for five full breath counts, working your way up to ten full breath counts.
- Return to your neutral position.

SEATED REVERSE PRAYER POSE | *DIFFICULTY—MEDIUM TO HARD (MEDIUM WITH MODIFICATION)*

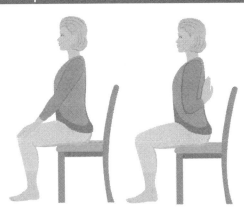

- Remain in your seated position, feet flat on the floor, and spine straight and tall.
- Shift your position slightly forward on your chair to make space for your hands behind your back.
- Once you are comfortable and balanced, inhale deeply and bring your hands together behind you at your lower back.
- Try to connect your hands together, facing upward towards your shoulders, in the prayer position.

- Bring focus to your breath.
- Hold this asana for five full breath counts.
- If you cannot point your hands up toward your shoulders, that is perfectly fine. Try to bring your hands together as close as possible, positioning them comfortably.
- Return to your neutral position.

Remember to remain seated in your neutral position for a few breath counts. Get up slowly from your work out and if you feel dizzy, remain seated until the feeling passes.

Targeted Exercises for Core and Abdominal Muscles

Having a strong core is absolutely vital for our health and well-being. These muscles play a critical role in supporting and stabilizing our bodies while we go about our day and get things done. Our core and abdominal muscles improve our posture, enhance our balance, reduce back pain, allow for functional movement like bending, lifting, and twisting, enhance our digestion and breathing, and even enhance our blood flow to our organs. These are the muscles that allow us to stand up straight and tall and allow us to perform everyday tasks with confidence.

Seniors can sometimes neglect these muscles citing back pain or opting to strengthen other muscles in their bodies, but the issue with having a weakened core is that no matter how strong our other muscles are, our balance and stability become compromised. As with the asanas provided in the previous sections, feel free to modify these to suit your specific limitations or comfort levels until you are able to complete them without pain.

SEATED ARDHA MATSYENDRASANA–SEATED SPINAL TWIST | *DIFFICULTY–EASY*

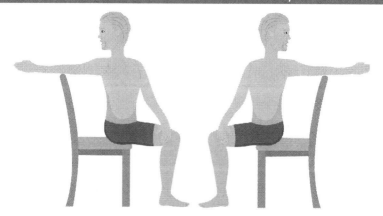

- Sit comfortably on your chair, spine tall and stretched and feet flat on the floor, hip-width apart—this is your neutral position.
- Inhale and length your spine toward the ceiling.

- Bring focus to your breath.
- As you begin to exhale, slowly twist your torso to the right.
- Lift your left hand and place it on your right knee.
- Engage your core by tightening your belly muscles as best you can.
- Slowly, lift your right hand up toward your right side, elbow straight, and palm facing down toward the floor.
- Hold this pose for five full breath counts.
- Return to your neutral position.
- Now, bring focus to your breath.
- As you begin to exhale, slowly twist your torso to the left.
- Lift your right hand and place it on your left knee.
- Engage your core by tightening your belly muscles as best you can.
- Slowly, lift your left hand up toward your left side, elbow straight, and palm facing down toward the floor.
- Hold this pose for five full breath counts.
- Return to your neutral position.

SEATED BOAT ASANA | *DIFFICULTY—EASY TO MEDIUM*

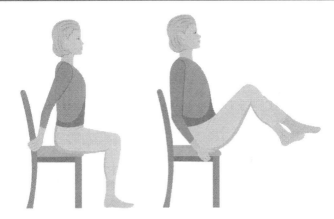

- Remain in your seated position, feet flat on the floor, and spine straight and tall.
- Place your hands on the side of your seating area for support.
- Bring focus to your breath.
- As you inhale, lift both feet off the floor, lifting them until you're a comfortable distance off the floor—2 to 4 inches.
- Balance on your sit bones and engage your core to lift your chest.
- Hold this position for five full breath counts, working your way up to eight full breath counts.
- Should you find this asana to be too easy, try lifting both arms up straight to your sides, palms facing down toward the floor.
- Return to your neutral position.

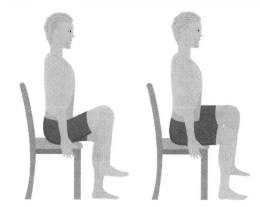

- Remain in your seated position, feet flat on the floor, and spine straight and tall.
- Place your hands on the side of your seating area for support.
- Bring focus to your breath.
- Inhale deeply and lift your right knee off the ground towards your chest.
- As you begin to exhale, engage your core and push your chest out, try to point your toes towards the ground.
- Do *not* sit back, try to keep your spine straight, shoulders relaxed, and pelvis straight and facing forward.
- Hold for five full breath counts.
- Return to your neutral position.
- Now, inhale deeply and lift your left knee off the ground towards your chest.
- As you begin to exhale, engage your core and push your chest out, try to point your toes towards the ground.
- Do *not* sit back, try to keep your spine straight, shoulders relaxed, and pelvis straight and facing forward.
- Hold for five full breath counts.
- Return to your neutral position.

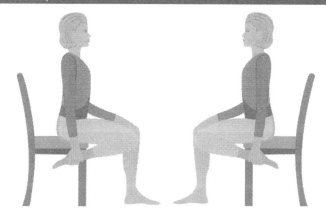

- Remain in your seated position, feet flat on the floor, and spine straight and tall.
- Place your hands on the side of your seating area for support.

- Bring focus to your breath and inhale deeply.
- As you exhale, slowly lift your right leg off the floor, keeping your knee bent.
- Lift your right hand off the seating area and try to grab hold of your right shin—if you can't grab hold of your shin, feel free to use a strap or towel around your shin to hold the pose.
- Hold this position for five full breath counts.
- Return to your neutral position.
- Bring focus back to your breath and inhale deeply.
- As you exhale, slowly lift your left leg off the floor, keeping your knee bent.
- Lift your left hand off the seating area and try to grab hold of your left shin—if you can't grab hold of your shin, feel free to use a strap or towel around your shin to hold the pose.
- Hold this position for five full breath counts.
- Return to your neutral position.

SEATED COBRA ASANA | DIFFICULTY EASY TO MEDIUM

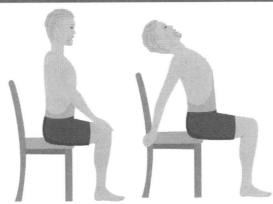

- Remain in your seated position, feet flat on the floor, and spine straight and tall.
- Place your hands on your thighs, palms facing down.
- Shift your seating slightly forward until you're about in the middle of your seating area—make sure your feet are firmly on the ground and that your chair won't tip forward.
- Bring focus to your breath and inhale deeply.
- Exhale and lift your hands from your thighs, slowly reaching back toward the backrest of your chair—if you cannot reach the backrest, feel free to use a long towel or strap around the back of the chair to complete the pose.
- Grasp the sides of the backrest firmly and push your chest out toward the ceiling.
- Slowly lift your head upward and engage your core.

- Hold this position for five full breath counts, working your way up to ten full breath counts.
- Release and return to your neutral position.

SEATED TRIANGLE ASANA | *DIFFICULTY EASY TO MEDIUM*

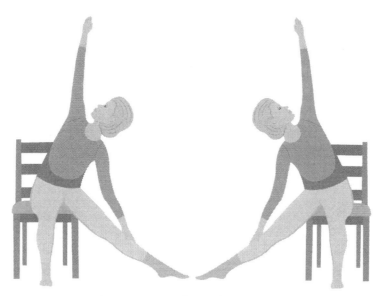

- Remain in your seated position, feet flat on the floor, and spine straight and tall.
- Place your hands on your thighs, palms facing down.
- Shift your seating slightly forward until you're about in the middle of your seating area—make sure your feet are firmly on the ground and that your chair won't tip forward.
- Lift your right thigh and move it toward your right side as wide as you comfortably can.
- Straighten your right leg.
- Now, straighten your left leg in front of you.
- Bring focus to your breath.
- Inhale deeply and lift your left arm above your head, keeping your elbow straight and your shoulders relaxed.
- As you exhale, slowly slide your right arm down your right leg—make sure you are not unbalanced and that your body is in a comfortable, manageable position, spine straight and core engaged.
- Hold for five full breath counts.
- Return to your neutral position.
- Lift your left thigh and move it toward your left side as wide as you comfortably can.
- Straighten your left leg.

- Now, straighten your right leg in front of you.
- Bring focus to your breath.
- Inhale deeply and lift your right arm above your head, keeping your elbow straight and your shoulders relaxed.
- As you exhale, slowly slide your left arm down your left leg—make sure you are not unbalanced and that your body is in a comfortable, manageable position, spine straight and core engaged.
- Hold for five full breath counts.
- Return to your neutral position.

SEATED BOAT POSE WITH STRAIGHT LEGS | *DIFFICULTY—HARD*

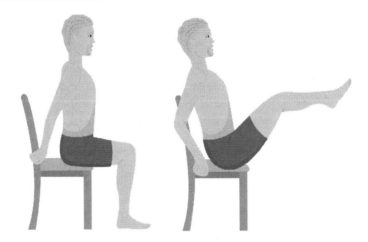

- Remain in your seated position, feet flat on the floor, and spine straight and tall.
- Place your hands on the sides of your seat on either side of your thighs.
- Shift your rear all the way forward until you are on the edge of your seat.
- Slide your feet forward until your legs are straight, knees and ankles touching.
- Lean your torso back until it touches your backrest.
- Make sure you are comfortable and balanced, adjusting your sit bones and hands appropriately.
- Bring focus to your breath and slowly lift both legs off the floor using your core muscles—if you cannot lift your legs just yet, that's perfectly fine, try to lift them until you feel your core engage and hold the position.
- Hold for three full breath counts, working your way up to eight full breath counts.
- Return to your neutral position and focus on your breath for three full breath counts before moving on to your next asana.

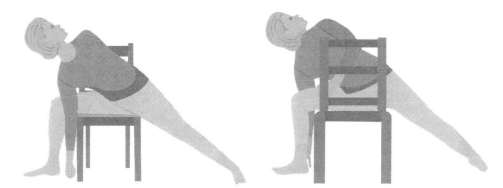

- Remain in your seated position, feet flat on the floor, and spine straight and tall.
- Now, shift slightly forward so that only half of your thighs are supported by the chair, and make sure you're comfortably balanced.
- Inhale deeply and lift your right leg up, opening it as wide as you can toward the right side of your chair—try to open your pelvis by tilting it forward slightly but be safe with your balance.
- Straighten your right leg, keeping your left leg bent—your legs should now be in a triangle shape with one leg straight and one leg bent.
- Bring focus to your breath and as you exhale, shift your right hand behind your back, resting it on your lower back.
- Engage your core and slide your left arm down your bent left leg, reaching for the floor—if you can, place your hand palm down flat on the ground.
- Keep your core engaged, spine straight, and feet firmly on the ground.
- Hold this pose for three full breath counts, working your way up to five full breath counts.
- Return to your neutral position, slightly forward on your chair, and half your thighs supported.
- Inhale deeply and lift your left leg up, opening it as wide as you can toward the left side of your chair—try to open your pelvis by tilting it forward slightly but be safe with your balance.
- Straighten your left leg, keeping your right leg bent—your legs should now be in a triangle shape with one leg straight and one leg bent.
- Bring focus to your breath and as you exhale, shift your left hand behind your back, resting it on your lower back.
- Engage your core and slide your right arm down your right left leg, reaching for the floor—if you can, place your hand palm down flat on the ground.
- Keep your core engaged, spine straight, and feet firmly on the ground.

- Hold this pose for three full breath counts, working your way up to five full breath counts.
- Return to your neutral position.

SEATED MARICHYASANA III–SEATED SIDE OBLIQUE ASANA | *DIFFICULTY–MEDIUM*

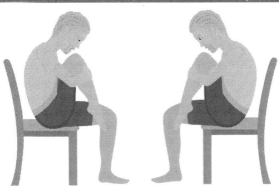

- Remain in your seated position, feet flat on the floor, and spine straight and tall.
- Place your hands on the side of your seating area for support.
- Bring focus to your breath.

- Inhale deeply and lift your right knee off the ground towards your chest, placing it on the seat if you can—if you cannot lift your foot all the way up to your seat, keep your foot on the ground, lifting your heel so that only the ball of your foot is touching the ground.
- As you exhale, twist your torso toward the right.
- Engage your core and lift both arms up to your sides, bringing them in towards your lifted knee in a sweeping motion.
- Using both your arms, hold onto your right bent knee as if you were hugging it.
- Keep your spine straight, inhale deeply, and engage your core.
- Hold this position for five full breath counts.
- Return to your neutral position.
- Bring focus to your breath.
- Inhale deeply and lift your left knee off the ground towards your chest, placing it on the seat if you can—if you cannot lift your foot all the way up to your seat, keep your foot on the ground, lifting your heel so that only the ball of your foot is touching the ground.
- As you exhale, twist your torso toward the left.
- Engage your core and lift both arms up to your sides, bringing them in towards your lifted knee in a sweeping motion.

- Using both your arms, hold onto your left bent knee as if you were hugging it.
- Keep your spine straight, inhale deeply, and engage your core.
- Hold this position for five full breath counts.
- Return to your neutral position.

HALF-SEATED BOAT ASANA | *DIFFICULTY MEDIUM TO HARD*

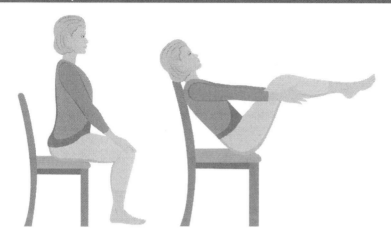

- Remain in your seated position, feet flat on the floor, and spine straight and tall.
- Place your hands on the side of your seating area for support.
- Bring focus to your breath.
- Inhale deeply and hold onto the sides of your chair.
- Lift both your bent knees up off the floor, trying to form a V-shape with your pelvis—if you cannot get into this position comfortably, lift your feet as high as you can.
- Lean back into your backrest but do not hunch your spine—if the pose is too easy for you, lift your hands off your seat and bring them out in front of you with straight arms.
- Hold this position for five full breath counts, working your way up to eight full breath counts.
- Return to your neutral position.

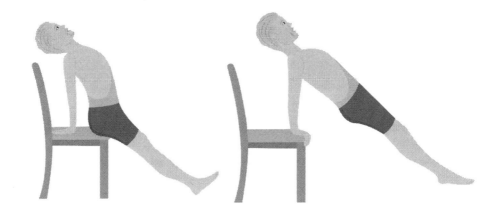

- Place your chair against a wall so that it cannot shift backward or tilt over.
- Remain in your seated position, feet flat on the floor, and spine straight and tall.
- Place your hands on the side of your seating area for support.
- Shift your rear all the way forward until half your glute cheeks are on the seating area.
- Straighten your legs out in front of you, big toes and knees touching and legs as straight as possible.
- Bring focus to your breath.
- Inhale deeply, engaging your core.
- As you exhale, lift your pelvis off the chair, straightening your body out as much as you possibly can—try to form a flat table top with your body. You can keep your elbows slightly bent if you feel your balance is off.
- Hold this position for three breath counts, working your way up to ten full breath counts.
- Carefully return to your neutral position by bending your elbows and shuffling your feet backward until your rear touches the seat again.

Remain seated in your neutral position for a few breath counts. Assess your balance and whether or not you feel dizzy after these workouts and give your body time to readjust before getting up.

Targeted Asanas for Legs

Strong, healthy legs are absolutely vital in our senior years. They're our mobility, our independence, and our ability to enjoy a quality life. As we age, however, we risk losing muscle mass and suffer from decreased bone density as sedentary habits and mobility issues creep in.

Having said that, we *can* still build strong legs in our senior years and improve our mobility, reduce our risk of falls, and improve bone health.

Strong legs have also been linked to improved cardiovascular health and back pain management and ensures we can maintain our active daily living tasks like bathing ourselves, getting our own shoes on, getting up from chairs and our bed, and so on.

The asanas in this section are designed to help us increase the strength and flexibility in our legs without the sometimes difficult traditional leg exercises like squats and lunges.

Feel free to modify these asanas to suit your specific limitations or comfort levels until you are able to complete them without pain.

SEATED BUTTERFLY ASANA | *DIFFICULTY–EASY TO MEDIUM*

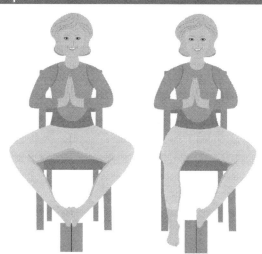

- Sit comfortably on your chair, spine tall and stretched and feet flat on the floor, hip-width apart—this is your neutral position.
- Inhale and length your spine toward the ceiling.
- Shift your rear forward in your seat.
- Place your hands on the sides of the chair to stabilize yourself.
- Bring the soles of your feet together, allowing your knees to drop out to the sides of your chair—try to have your feet touching at all points.
- Bring focus to your breath and inhale deeply.
- Lean forward, bending your torso at your hips until you feel stretching in your hamstrings and along your inner thighs.
- Exhale, and straighten your spine as much as you can.
- Hold this position for five breath counts, working your way up to ten full breath counts.
- Slowly return to your neutral position.

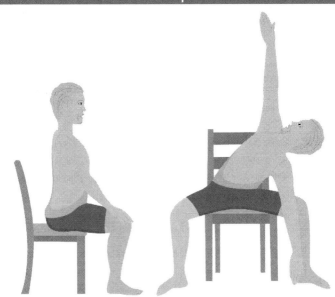

- Sit comfortably on your chair in your neutral position.
- Inhale and length your spine toward the ceiling.
- Shift your rear forward in your seat.
- Slowly separate your legs, moving them as wide as you can—do not straighten your legs, they should remain bent at the knee throughout this asana.
- Make sure your feet are firmly on the ground and that you have balance.
- Bring focus to your breath.
- Inhale and as you do, slowly lift your right hand to the ceiling.
- As you exhale, slowly bend your torso forward from the hips, bringing your right arm down to meet your right ankle.
- If you can, place your hand on the floor, or for a deeper stretch, hold your ankle and pull down, being careful to maintain your balance.
- Hold for five full breath counts.
- Return to your neutral position.
- Once more, inhale and length your spine toward the ceiling.
- Shift your rear forward in your seat.
- Slowly separate your legs, moving them as wide as you can—do not straighten your legs, they should remain bent at the knee throughout this asana.
- Make sure your feet are firmly on the ground and that you have balance.
- Bring focus to your breath.
- Inhale and as you do, slowly lift your left hand to the ceiling.
- As you exhale, slowly bend your torso forward from the hips, bringing your left arm down to meet your left ankle.
- If you can, place your hand on the floor, or for a deeper stretch, hold your ankle and pull down, being careful to maintain your balance.

- Hold for five full breath counts.
- Return to your neutral position.

JANU SIRSASANA–DEEP HAMSTRING STRETCH ASANA | *DIFFICULTY–EASY*

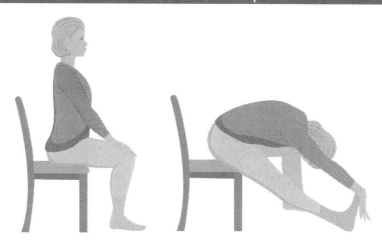

- Sit comfortably on your chair in your neutral position.
- Inhale and length your spine toward the ceiling.
- Extend your right leg out in front of you, keeping your foot on the floor but your knee straight. Your left leg remains bent and firmly on the floor.
- Bring focus to your breath and inhale deeply as you reach up toward the ceiling with both arms.
- As you exhale, lean forward, bending at your hips, and bring your arms down over your head toward your outstretched right leg.
- If you can, hold your ankle–if you can't reach your ankle, feel free to use a towel or strap to help you get into the pose. Alternatively, you can try moving forward on your seat to help deepen your stretch.
- Make sure you're not putting too much strain on your hamstring. You should feel a slight, but comfortable stretch or pull.
- Hold this position for five breath counts, working your way up to eight full breath counts.
- Carefully return to your neutral position.
- Extend your left leg out in front of you, keeping your foot on the floor but your knee straight. Your right leg remains bent and firmly on the floor.
- Bring focus to your breath again.
- Inhale deeply as you reach up toward the ceiling with both arms.
- As you exhale, lean forward, bending at your hips, and bring your arms down over your head toward your outstretched left leg.
- If you can, hold your ankle–if you can't reach your ankle, feel free to use a towel or strap to help you get into the pose. Alternatively, you can try moving forward on your seat to help deepen your stretch.

- Make sure you're not putting too much strain on your hamstring. You should feel a slight, but comfortable stretch or pull.
- Hold this position for five breath counts, working your way up to eight full breath counts.
- Carefully return to your neutral position.

FIGURE OF FOUR ASANA | *DIFFICULTY–MEDIUM TO HARD*

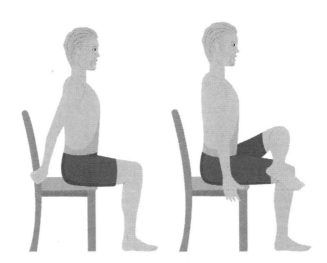

- Sit comfortably on your chair in your neutral position.
- Inhale and length your spine toward the ceiling.
- Shift forward on your seat until about half of your thighs are on the chair.
- Drop your arms down to your sides, or hold onto the side of the chair if you're unsure of your balance.
- Lift your right leg up to your left thigh in a crossed-leg position—aim to have your right ankle placed in the center of your left thigh if possible. If you cannot lift your leg to this position, feel free to use a towel or strap to lift it as high as possible without strain or discomfort.
- Bring focus to your breath and as you exhale, bring your arms up to the center of your chest, palms together in a prayer position.
- Hold this asana for five full breath counts—to deepen the stretch you can lean forward slightly, bending from your hips.
- Return to your neutral position.
- Shift forward on your seat once more until about half your thighs are on the chair.
- Drop your arms down to your sides, or hold onto the side of the chair if you're unsure of your balance.
- Lift your left leg up to your right thigh in a crossed-leg position—aim to have your left ankle placed in the center of your right thigh if possible. If you cannot

lift your leg to this position, feel free to use a towel or strap to lift it as high as possible without strain or discomfort.

- Bring focus to your breath and as you exhale, bring your arms up to the center of your chest, palms together in a prayer position.
- Hold this asana for five full breath counts—to deepen the stretch you can lean forward slightly, bending from your hips.
- Return to your neutral position.

SEATED DEEP QUAD STRETCH | *DIFFICULTY–MEDIUM TO HARD*

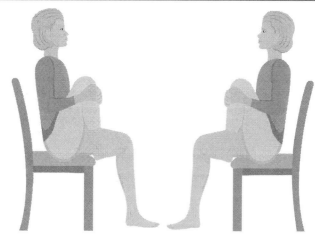

- Sit comfortably on your chair in your neutral position.
- Inhale and length your spine toward the ceiling.
- Place your hands on your thighs, palms down, or for additional balance, place your hands on the sides of your seat.
- Bring focus to your breath.
- On your exhale, raise your right foot off the floor, lifting your thigh up and towards your chest.
- When you feel the stretch, stop and hold the position for five full breath counts—if you cannot support the weight of your leg just yet, feel free to use a towel or strap to help lift your leg.
- Return to your neutral position.
- Now, return focus to your breath.
- On your exhale, raise your left foot off the floor, lifting your thigh up and towards your chest.
- When you feel the stretch, stop and hold the position for five full breath counts—if you cannot support the weight of your leg just yet, feel free to use a towel or strap to help lift your leg.
- Return to your neutral position.

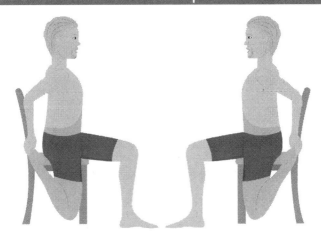

- Sit comfortably on your chair in your neutral position.
- Shift your body forward so that three-quarters of your thighs are on your seat and the remainder of your thighs are off the seat, supported by your feet.
- Inhale and length your spine toward the ceiling.
- Keeping your left leg bent at the knee and your foot firmly on the ground, lift and bend your right leg back towards your rear—if you like, you can hold your leg with your right hand, or alternatively, use a towel or strap to support your leg's weight.
- Your right leg should now form a V-shape.
- Exhale deeply and hold this position for five full breath counts—to deepen the stretch you can lean forward slightly, bending at your hips. Pay special attention to your balance and don't lean too far forward.
- Gently bring your right leg to the floor and return to your neutral position.
- Bring focus to your breath again.
- This time, keep your right leg bent at the knee and your foot firmly on the ground and lift and bend your left leg back towards your rear—if you like, you can hold your leg with your left hand, or alternatively, use a towel or strap to support your leg's weight.
- Your left leg should now form a V-shape.
- Exhale deeply and hold this position for five full breath counts—to deepen the stretch you can lean forward slightly, bending at your hips. Pay special attention to your balance and don't lean too far forward.
- Gently bring your left leg to the floor and return to your neutral position.

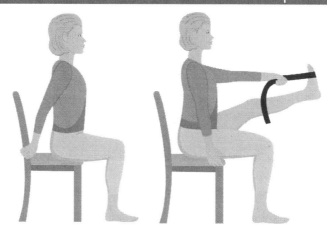

This asana requires a towel or a strap to complete.

- Sit comfortably on your chair in your neutral position.
- Shift your body forward so that half of your thighs are on your seat and the remainder of your thighs are off the seat, supported by your feet.
- Wrap your strap or towel around the center of your right foot, with the ends of the towel being held in each of your hands.
- Inhale and length your spine toward the ceiling as much as possible.
- Bring your focus to your breath.
- On your exhale, slowly lean back on your chair, lifting your right foot off the floor.
- Straighten your right leg as much as possible, using the towel or strap as balance and support.
- Hold this position for five full breath counts, working your way up to eight full breath counts.
- Slowly lower your right leg back to the floor and return to your neutral position.
- Wrap your strap or towel around the center of your left foot, with the ends of the towel being held in each of your hands.
- Inhale and length your spine toward the ceiling as much as possible.
- Bring your focus to your breath.
- On your exhale, slowly lean back on your chair, lifting your left foot off the floor.
- Straighten your left leg as much as possible, using the towel or strap as balance and support.
- Hold this position for five full breath counts, working your way up to eight full breath counts.
- Slowly lower your left leg back to the floor and return to your neutral position.

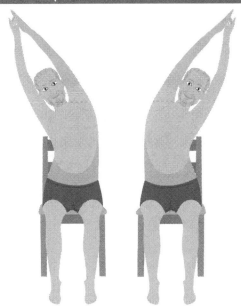

- Sit comfortably on your chair in your neutral position.
- Make sure your back is against the backrest of the chair and that your spine is straight.
- Bring focus to your breath.
- Inhale deeply and lift your arms above your head, keep your elbows slightly bent, and place your palms together in the prayer position.
- On your exhale, bend your torso slightly to the right so that your upper body forms a crescent moon shape.
- On your next inhale, lift your right leg out straight in front of you—concentrate on your balance. If you feel you're going to tip, drop your left arm and hold the side of your seat for support.
- Hold this position for five full breath counts, working your way up to eight full breath counts.
- Slowly return to your neutral position.
- Bring focus to your breath once more.
- Inhale deeply and lift your arms above your head, keep your elbows slightly bent, and place your palms together in the prayer position.
- On your exhale, bend your torso slightly to the left so that your upper body forms a crescent moon shape.
- On your next inhale, lift your left leg out straight in front of you—concentrate on your balance. If you feel you're going to tip, drop your right arm and hold the side of your seat for support.
- Hold this position for five full breath counts, working your way up to eight full breath counts.
- Slowly return to your neutral position.

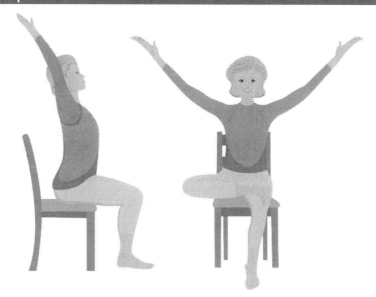

- Sit comfortably on your chair in your neutral position.
- Make sure your back is against the backrest of the chair and that your spine is straight.
- Bring focus to your breath.
- Slowly lift your right foot up off the floor—depending on your strength level you can leave your foot hanging off the floor, or lift it all the way up, resting it on your left thigh.
- As you exhale, slowly lift both of your arms above your head. Keep your arms straight, hands pointed towards the ceiling, open slightly in a V-shape.
- Slowly lean your body forward, bending at the hips until you feel the stretch on your upper legs and inner thighs.
- Hold this position for five full breath counts.
- Return to your neutral position.
- Slowly lift your left foot up off the floor—depending on your strength level you can leave your foot hanging off the floor, or lift it all the way up, resting it on your right thigh.
- As you exhale, slowly lift both of your arms above your head. Keep your arms straight, hands pointed towards the ceiling, open slightly in a V-shape.
- Slowly lean your body forward, bending at the hips until you feel the stretch on your upper legs and inner thighs.
- Hold this position for five full breath counts.
- Return to your neutral position.

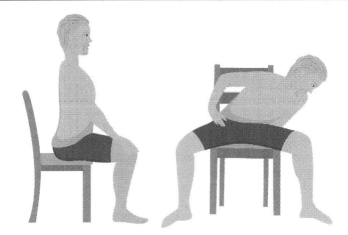

- Sit comfortably on your chair in your neutral position.
- Shift your position slightly forward so that three-quarters of your thighs are on the seat and the other quarter is off your chair and supported by your feet.
- Open your legs as wide as they will go but make sure your feet remain flat on the floor and that your balance is stable.
- Bring focus to your breath.
- On your inhale, lift your arms above your head, straightening your spine upwards.
- On your exhale, bend your torso forward from the hips, leaning slightly to your right knee.
- Hold this position for a count of five breaths.
- Do *not* return to your neutral position. Instead, slowly sweep your body from right to left.
- Hold this position for five breaths.
- This time, sweep your body to the right and repeat this movement five times or for 10 full breath counts in total.

Take the time after these asanas to remain seated, allowing your body to readjust and your legs to regain their strength.

Cool-Down Stretches

Cooling down after any workout, regardless of how gentle it is, is important to help our bodies transition from a state of increased activity to a resting state. When we cool down we allow our heart rate to gradually recover, reduce lactic acid pooling in our muscles, prevent blood pooling in our legs, and help begin the muscle repair and growth process.

Every workout should include both a warm-up and cool-down period so make sure that you end each of your full workouts, regardless of what they are, with cool-down stretches.

SEATED HEART OPENER | *DIFFICULTY—EASY*

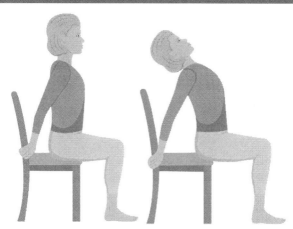

- Sit comfortably on your chair, spine tall and stretched and feet flat on the floor—this is your neutral position.
- Shift slightly on your seat so that you have enough space to place your hands behind your back.
- Inhale deeply and straighten your spine toward the ceiling.
- Bring focus on your breath.
- On your exhale, bring your hands behind your back—interlink your hands if you can. If you can't, place your hands on your lower back, palms facing outward.
- Inhale deeply and open your chest, squeezing your shoulder blades together—to deepen the stretch you can lift your head up towards the ceiling.
- Hold this position for five full breath counts.
- This stretch should be gentle and not place strain on your body. Remember that these are not active stretches per sé. Rather, they're designed to gently release your muscles.
- Return to your neutral position.

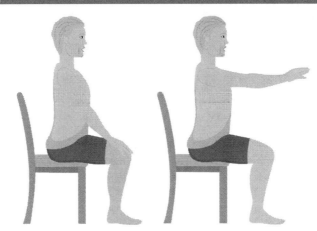

- Sit comfortably on your chair, spine tall and stretched and feet flat on the floor.
- Bring focus to your breath.
- On your inhale, lift your arms straight out in front of you to chest height.
- As you exhale, begin to roll your wrists—the direction of the roll isn't important, do what is comfortable for you.
- Complete rotations of your wrist ten times.
- Return to your neutral positions, hands on your thighs, palms down.

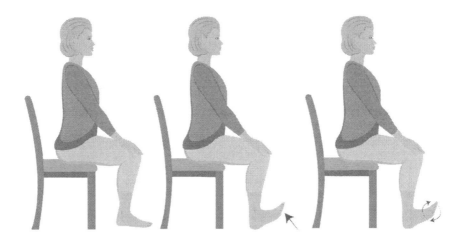

- Sit comfortably on your chair, spine tall and stretched and feet flat on the floor.
- Bring focus to your breath.
- On your exhale, lift your right foot off the floor ever so slightly—allow your toes to still touch the floor.
- Begin to roll your ankle—the direction of the roll isn't important, do what is comfortable for you.
- Complete rotations of your ankle ten times.

- Return to your neutral position.
- Bring focus to your breath.
- On your exhale, lift your left foot off the floor ever so slightly—allow your toes to still touch the floor.
- Begin to roll your ankle—the direction of the roll isn't important, do what is comfortable for you.
- Complete rotations of your ankle ten times.
- Return to your neutral position.

SEATED NECK ROLLS | *DIFFICULTY—EASY*

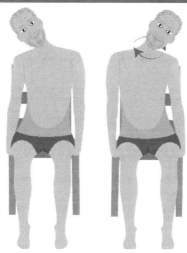

- Sit comfortably on your chair, spine tall and stretched and feet flat on the floor.
- Bring focus to your breath.
- On your inhale, lift your head up towards the ceiling.
- As you exhale, begin to roll your head from right to left—keep your movements controlled and slow.
- Complete five rotations.
- Return to your neutral position.
- Now, bring focus to your breath once more.
- On your inhale, lift your head up towards the ceiling.
- As you exhale, begin to roll your head from left to right—keep your movements controlled and slow.
- Complete five rotations.
- Return to your neutral position.

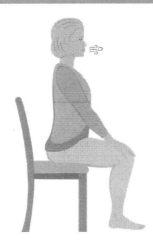

- Sit comfortably on your chair, spine tall and stretched and feet flat on the floor.
- Bring focus to your breath.
- Fix your gaze on a spot in the room—do not close your eyes.
- Place your hands on your thighs, palms down.
- Take a deep breath in through your nose, filling your lungs with oxygen.
- Hold this breath for a count of two.
- Exhale deeply through your mouth, emptying your body of all its carbon dioxide.
- Repeat this for five full breath counts.
- Return to your neutral position.

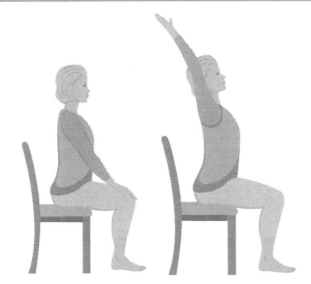

- Sit comfortably on your chair, spine tall and stretched and feet flat on the floor.
- Bring focus to your breath.

70

- As you inhale, slowly lift your hands above your head.
- Keep your arms straight and try to reach for the ceiling.
- On your exhale, slowly lean forward from the hips, sweeping your arms down towards the ground.
- On your next inhale, slowly lift your hands above your head once more, keeping your arms straight and reaching for the ceiling.
- Exhale, sweeping your arms down towards the floor once more.
- Complete three breaths this way, making sure to pay attention to gentle sweeping movements.
- Bring your hands to your chest, placing them in a prayer position, and give thanks to your body for its strength and flexibility.

Chapter 4
4-WEEK CHAIR YOGA PLAN WITH FREE GIFT

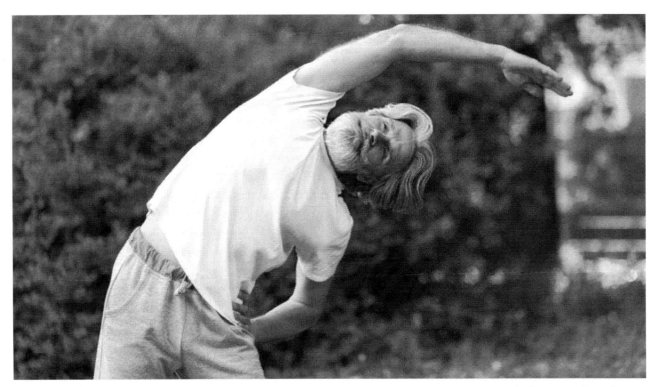

Now that we have the step-by-step instructions we need for each of our warm-up stretches, yoga asanas, and cool-down stretches, it's time to put all of this information together into a comprehensive, easy-to-follow plan.

The tables below are broken down into weeks that will incorporate all of the 50-featured exercises, the page of the exercise for ease of reference, and how many breath counts or reps need to be completed. But, don't stop reading once you've skimmed through these exercises!

This chapter contains an amazing free gift that will help you to monitor your progress, and celebrate your achievements.

Week-by-Week Chair Workout Plan

Before beginning each of the workouts planned for you below, complete each of the warm-up exercises—these are vital to prevent muscle strains and injury.

WEEK 1: KICKING OFF YOUR YOGA JOURNEY

Day 1

Asana/Stretch	Page	Repetitions
Tadasana–Seated Mountain Pose for Arms	33	3 to 10 breath counts: fitness dependant
Seated Shoulder Opener With Forward Fold	40	5 breath counts
Seated Paschimottanasana With Chest Opening Asana	42	3 to 5 breath counts: fitness dependant
Seated Ardha Matsyendrasana–Seated Spinal Twist	47	5 breath counts
Seated Wide-Leg Asana With Side Stretch	58	5 breath counts on either side

Day 2

Asana/Stretch	Page	Repetitions
Parivrtta Ardha Chandrasana–Seated Side Bend Asana	36	5 breath counts on either side
Seated Child's Pose	43	5 to 8 breath counts
Seated Prayer Twist	45	5 breath counts
Seated Knee Raise Asana	49	5 breath counts on either side
Janu Sirsasana–Deep Hamstring Stretch Asana	59	5 to 8 breath counts on either side

Day 3

Asana/Stretch	Page	Repetitions
Seated Chest Opening Asana	37	5 breath counts
Seated Boat Asana	48	5 breath counts
Seated Cobra Asana	50	5 to 10 breath counts: fitness dependant
Seated Half-Moon With Leg Lift	64	5 to 8 breath counts on each side: fitness dependant
Utthita Parsvakonasana–Extended Side Angle Asana	53	3 to 5 breath counts on each side: fitness dependant

Day 4		
Tadasana–Seated Mountain Pose for Arms	33	3 to 10 breath counts: fitness dependant
Seated Shoulder Blade Squeeze	46	5 to 10 breath counts
Seated Triangle Asana	51	5 breath counts on either side
Seated Ardha Matsyendrasana–Seated Spinal Twist	47	5 breath counts
Seated Butterfly Asana	57	5 to 10 breath counts: fitness dependant
Day 5		
Parivrtta Ardha Chandrasana–Seated Side Bend Asana	36	5 breath counts on either side
Seated Child's Pose	43	5 to 8 breath counts
Seated Cobra Asana	50	5 to 10 breath counts: fitness dependant
Seated Triangle Asana	51	5 breath counts on either side
Janu Sirsasana–Deep Hamstring Stretch Asana	59	5 to 8 breath counts on either side
Day 6		
Rest		

WEEK 2: GAINING STRENGTH

Day 7

Asana/Stretch	Page	Repetitions
Garudasana Arms–Seated Eagle Arms	33	3 to 10 breath counts: fitness dependant
Seated Chest Opening Asana	37	5 breath counts
Seated One Arm Twist	41	5 breath counts on either side
Seated Marichyasana III–Seated Side Oblique Asana	54	5 breath counts on either side
Seated Tree Asana	65	5 breath counts on either side

Day 8

Asana/Stretch	Page	Repetitions
Paschimottanasana–Seated Forward Bend Asana	35	3 to 8 breath counts: fitness dependant
Seated Ustrana–Camel Asana	43	5 to 8 breath counts
Seated Shoulder Blade Squeeze	46	5 to 10 breath counts
Seated Boat Asana	48	5 breath counts
Sweeping Circles Hip Opener	66	5 breaths

Day 9

Asana/Stretch	Page	Repetitions
Tadasana–Seated Mountain Pose for Arms	33	3 to 10 breath counts: fitness dependant
Seated Shoulder Press Asana	44	5 to 10 repetitions: fitness dependant
Seated Ardha Matsyendrasana–Seated Spinal Twist	47	5 breath counts
Seated Triangle Asana	51	5 breath counts on either side
Janu Sirsasana–Deep Hamstring Stretch Asana	59	5 to 8 breath counts on either side

Day 10		
Parivrtta Ardha Chandrasana–Seated Side Bend Asana	36	5 breath counts on either side
Seated Shoulder Opener With Forward Fold	40	5 breath counts
Seated Knee Raise Asana	49	5 breath counts on either side
Utthita Parsvakonasana–Extended Side Angle Asana	53	3 to 5 breath counts on each side: fitness dependant
Seated Butterfly Asana	57	5 to 10 breath counts: fitness dependant
Day 11		
Seated Cat-Cow Stretch	37	5 breath counts
Garudasana Arms–Seated Eagle Arms	33	3 to 10 breath counts: fitness dependant
Seated Child's Pose	43	5 to 8 breath counts
Seated Cobra Asana	50	5 to 10 breath counts: fitness dependant
Seated Wide-Leg Asana With Side Stretch	58	5 breath counts on either side
Day 12		
Rest		

Day 13

Asana/Stretch	Page	Repetitions
Paschimottanasana–Seated Forward Bend Asana	35	3 to 8 breath counts: fitness dependant
Seated Ustrana–Camel Asana	43	5 to 8 breath counts
Seated Ardha Matsyendrasana–Seated Spinal Twist	47	5 breath counts
Half-Seated Boat Asana	55	5 to 8 breath counts: fitness dependant
Seated Deep Quad Stretch	61	5 breath counts

Day 14

Parivrtta Ardha Chandrasana–Seated Side Bend Asana	36	5 breath counts on either side
Seated Shoulder Press Asana	44	5 to 10 repetitions: fitness dependant
Utthita Parsvakonasana–Extended Side Angle Asana	53	3 to 5 breath counts on each side: fitness dependant
Seated Shin Hold Asana	49	5 breath counts on each side
Figure of Four Asana	60	5 breath counts on each side

Day 15

Tadasana–Seated Mountain Pose for Arms	33	3 to 10 breath counts: fitness dependant
Seated Paschimottanasana With Chest Opening Asana	42	3 to 5 breath counts: fitness dependant
Seated Prayer Twist	45	5 breath counts
Seated Half-Moon With Leg Lift	64	5 to 8 breath counts on each side: fitness dependant
Seated Tree Asana	65	5 breath counts on either side

Day 16		
Seated Chest Expansion Asana	39	5 breath counts
Garudasana Arms–Seated Eagle Arms	33	3 to 10 breath counts: fitness dependant
Seated Shoulder Blade Squeeze	46	5 to 10 breath counts
Seated Triangle Asana	51	5 breath counts on either side
Virasana Hero's Pose–Seated Quad Stretch	62	5 breath counts on each side
Day 17		
Gomukhasana Arms–Seated Cow Face Arms Asana	34	3 breath counts on each side
Seated Cat-Cow Stretch	37	5 breath counts
Seated Shoulder Opener With Forward Fold	40	5 breath counts
Seated Cobra Asana	50	5 to 10 breath counts: fitness dependant
Janu Sirsasana–Deep Hamstring Stretch Asana	59	5 to 8 breath counts on either side
Day 18		
Rest		

WEEK 4: STRONG AND FLEXIBLE

Day 19

Asana/Stretch	Page	Repetitions
Seated Ardha Matsyendrasana–Seated Spinal Twist	47	5 breath counts
Seated Shoulder Press Asana	44	5 to 10 repetitions: fitness dependant
Seated Reverse Prayer Pose	46	5 breaths
Seated Marichyasana III–Seated Side Oblique Asana	54	5 breath counts on either side
Figure of Four Asana	60	5 breath counts on each side

Day 20

Seated Ustrana–Camel Asana	43	5 to 8 breath counts
Seated Child's Pose	43	5 to 8 breath counts
Seated Boat Pose With Straight Legs	52	3 to 8 breath counts: fitness dependant
Seated Cobra Asana	50	5 to 10 breath counts: fitness dependant
Seated Tree Asana	65	5 breath counts on either side

Day 21

Tadasana–Seated Mountain Pose for Arms	33	3 to 10 breath counts: fitness dependant
Seated Paschimottanasana With Chest Opening Asana	42	3 to 5 breath counts: fitness dependant
Seated Shin Hold Asana	50	5 breath counts on each side
Figure of Four Asana	60	5 breath counts on each side
Seated Deep Quad Stretch	61	5 breath counts

Day 22		
Seated Prayer Twist	45	5 breath counts
Seated One Arm Twist	41	5 breath counts on each side
Seated Shoulder Blade Squeeze	46	5 to 10 breath counts
Utthita Parsvakonasana–Extended Side Angle Asana	53	3 to 5 breath counts on each side: fitness dependant
Sweeping Circles Hip Opener	66	5 breaths
Day 23		
Seated Chest Expansion Asana	39	5 breath counts
Seated Shoulder Opener With Forward Fold	40	5 breath counts
Seated Child's Pose	43	5 to 8 breath counts
Upward Plank Pose	56	3 to 10 breath counts: fitness dependant
Utthita Hasta Padangustasana–Seated Full Leg Stretch	63	5 to 8 breath counts: fitness dependant
Day 24		
Rest		

Day 25

Asana/Stretch	Page	Repetitions
Figure of Four Asana	60	5 breath counts on each side
Seated Triangle Asana	51	5 breath counts on either side
Seated Shoulder Blade Squeeze	46	5 to 10 breath counts
Seated Shoulder Opener With Forward Fold	40	5 breath counts
Seated Ardha Matsyendrasana–Seated Spinal Twist	47	5 breath counts

Day 26

Janu Sirsasana–Deep Hamstring Stretch Asana	59	5 to 8 breath counts on either side
Seated Shoulder Press Asana	44	5 to 10 repetitions: fitness dependant
Parivrtta Ardha Chandrasana–Seated Side Bend Asana	36	5 breath counts on either side
Seated Tree Asana	65	5 breath counts on either side
Tadasana–Seated Mountain Pose for Arms	33	3 to 10 breath counts: fitness dependant

Day 27

Janu Sirsasana–Deep Hamstring Stretch Asana	59	5 to 8 breath counts on either side
Seated Child's Pose	43	5 to 8 breath counts
Seated Paschimottanasana With Chest Opening Asana	42	3 to 5 breath counts: fitness dependant
Seated Half-Moon With Leg Lift	64	5 to 8 breath counts on each side: fitness dependant
Seated Butterfly Asana	57	5 to 10 breath counts: fitness dependant

Day 28		
Seated Cobra Asana	50	5 to 10 breath counts: fitness dependant
Seated One Arm Twist	41	5 breath counts on each side
Virasana Hero's Pose–Seated Quad Stretch	62	5 breath counts on each side
Garudasana Arms–Seated Eagle Arms	33	3 to 10 breath counts: fitness dependant
Seated Knee Raise Asana	49	5 breath counts on either side
Day 29		
Seated Marichyasana III–Seated Side Oblique Asana	54	5 breath counts on either side
Utthita Hasta Padangustasana–Seated Full Leg Stretch	63	5 to 8 breath counts: fitness dependant
Seated Cat-Cow Stretch	37	5 breath counts
Seated Shin Hold Asana	49	5 breath counts on each side
Upward Plank Pose	56	3 to 10 breath counts: fitness dependant
Day 30		
Rest		

Monitoring Your Progress and Celebrating Your Achievements

When we make changes to our lives that benefit our mental and physical well-being it can be challenging. We know that what we're doing is for the better but old habits die hard, and we can become so lost in the struggle that we can forget our goals altogether.

Motivation is great, really it is—we all have it and it's what we need to get out of the starting blocks when it comes to taking on new tasks.

But, motivation is temporary and at some point, it gives way to self-discipline, or a lack thereof.

We need to be able to encourage ourselves as we face the inevitable challenges life gives us and overcome these challenges, and slowly build our self-confidence.

We need to be able to set achievable, meaningful goals that can be fine-tuned and adjusted as we reach each of our milestones, and we need a solid way to track our health improvements without heading off to the resident nurse or our health practitioner.

We can monitor our plateaus, uncover our setbacks, and create a journey out of our health and our lives in which we're firmly in the driver's seat rather than being a passenger on a bus to aging degradation. And rather than accepting our fate, we learn to create accountability for the things we can do while acknowledging the things we can't.

We enhance our ability to commit long-term to our health and well-being by activating the reward system in our brains and reinforcing that all of these changes bring us joy.

For many seniors, effectively monitoring progress and success is the final hurdle that just cannot be overcome because they have no way of actively tracking just how strong they are becoming.

They live in a time that is not understanding that our senior years are the best time for a "great reset" and that our journey should begin on a fresh page—not in a book that has already been written.

And it's this new book, fresh page, and celebration that I want to share with you. Below, you'll find a QR code that can be scanned for your free, downloadable, and printable copy of the *ForeverFit Progress Journal*.

With this journal as your aid and guide you can renew your motivation, build self-discipline, actively track your progress, and celebrate all of your fitness and wellness achievements.

When using this journal you will be able to look back on where you have started so that you can begin to uncover where you are succeeding—and what might need a little extra work—and identify possible patterns in the challenges you are facing.

Once challenges are identified they can be overcome, goals can be finetuned and you can return your focus to the task at hand—creating a strong, flexible, senior body.

So, with all of this in mind, and with your workout plan in hand, our final step is to take care of our senior nutrition so that we can nourish our bodies and minds as we move forward into a new era of health and wellness.

SCAN ME

Chapter 5

THE POWER OF NUTRITION IN WEIGHT LOSS

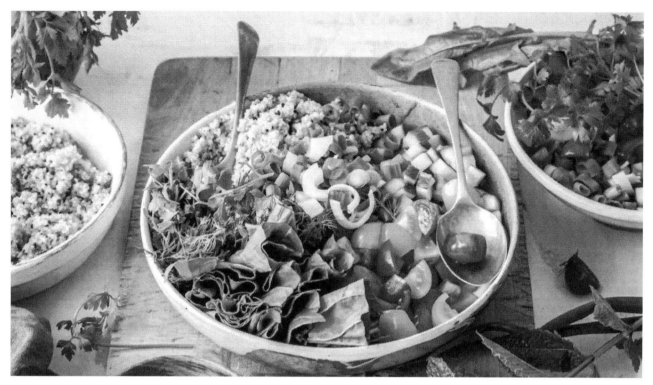

Nutrition plays a role in our health throughout our lives but as we get older we realize that the double cheeseburger and extra-large soda aren't going to miraculously disappear from our waistline and that making healthy food choices can play a pretty significant role in our ability to maintain and lose weight.

Our appetites may begin to change, certain foods we once loved are no longer appealing, and we may find that we are inexplicably picking up weight. Now we've already dispelled the myth that *active* seniors do not require substantially fewer calories, but it's still important to understand that we need to eat a caloric-balanced diet.

Weight loss relies on us eating in a calorie deficit but we still need to eat the right nutrition to make sure that the calories we are taking in count toward our feelings of fullness as well as our health. Another thing to keep in mind is that the types of food we eat can influence our metabolism. Protein-rich foods will help boost metabolism because they take more energy to digest while simple carbs digest without much energy expenditure at all.

Certain foods will help us remain fuller for longer and stabilize our blood sugar levels and fiber-rich fruits and vegetables are definitely going to help keep our hunger at bay a lot better than sugar-laden snacks.

But, the reality is that you're going to need to make some adjustments when it comes to your diet if you're hoping to lose *fat*. Now you'll notice that the previous sentence says lose fat and not weight and there's a good reason for that.

Weight is exactly that—weight—whether muscle or fat, it's still weight. Muscle is great for our metabolism and for our strength and health but fat is unhealthy and causes a number of chronic diseases as well as joint pain, inflammation, and increases our risk of heart attack and stroke. What we need to aim for is to lose fat, not weight, and the reality is that we absolutely cannot exercise away a *bad* diet.

We need to eat a diet that supports our physical activity so that we can fuel our bodies correctly and if need be, create a healthy calorie deficit with physical activity. Okay, so how do we create this nutritious, satiating diet so that we can fuel our bodies correctly while exercising?

1. We need to prioritize nutrient-dense foods like lean proteins, fruits and vegetables, whole grains, and healthy fats in fatty fish, avocados, nuts, seeds, and so on.
2. We should be mindful of how much we're eating and seek to control our portion sizes.
3. We can't slack on the water—hunger can easily be mistaken for thirst.
4. We need to stay away from processed, high-fat foods and snacks.
5. We should stay away from sugary beverages.
6. We need to become mindful when we eat, paying attention to our body's natural cues that tell us we're full.

Seniors do, however, have very specific dietary needs that we need to be mindful of. Our protein, calcium, vitamin D, and fiber requirements all need adjustment as we enter our senior years.

Now, don't worry, the final chapter of this book will help you to adjust your diet and supply you with recipes, a meal plan, and a shopping list so that this process is a lot easier to include in your life. For now, let's focus on the nutrition you do need.

- Protein is vitally important for supporting and maintaining muscle mass and strength. As we age, we tend to become more sedentary and our appetite may have us turn away from animal forms of protein. However, protein can be found in a whole lot of foods including fish, beans, tofu, eggs, legumes, dairy, seeds, and nuts.
- Calcium and vitamin D are essential for bone health and in preventing degenerative bone diseases. Calcium and vitamin D can be eaten in dairy, fortified grains and plant milk, leafy green vegetables, canned fish, cereals, and dietary supplements. The greatest source of vitamin D we have is sunlight

and getting outdoors for just 10 minutes every day can supply our bodies with all the vitamin D it needs.

- As we age, we may find it more difficult to absorb vitamin B12 in the foods we eat. Having said that, we need vitamin B12 to facilitate red blood cell production and make sure our nerve health is great. B12 can be obtained from fortified foods, animal products, and supplementation.
- Fiber helps to keep our stomach regular and feeds the good bacteria in our gut so that we can synthesize the right vitamins and minerals we need. Thankfully, good sources of fiber are available to us in all fruits and vegetables as well as in nuts, seeds, and beans.
- Our bodies require healthy fats to help support brain function and reduce inflammation in our bodies. These fats should be limited to those found in nuts, seeds, avocados, and fatty fish and seniors should stay away from trans fats that are found in processed and deep-fried foods.
- Potassium and magnesium help support heart health, regulate blood pressure as well as facilitating muscle and nerve function as well as bone health. Potassium and magnesium can be found in tomatoes, oranges, bananas, leafy greens, nuts, seeds, and whole grains.
- Vitamin C and other antioxidants help to improve our immune system by ridding our bodies of excess free radicals. Added to this, vitamin C is important for our skin health and supports our overall health. These two elements can be found in fruits and vegetables like oranges, berries, kiwi fruit, peppers, and colorful vegetables.
- Finally, omega-3 fatty acids are essential for our heart and brain health and help keep us energized and focused throughout the day. These fatty acids can be found in seeds, fatty fish, and nuts—more specifically walnuts.

How to Make Smart Good Choices For Optimal Health and Weight Loss

We know that we need to prioritize a healthy, balanced diet that includes a wide range of nutrient-dense foods but sometimes we can get lost in the convenience of putting a microwave meal on and sitting in front of the television to eat.

Here's the thing about these processed, fast foods. Even if they don't come from a drive-through window, chances are they're salt and chemical-laden and just aren't great for our bodies.

Making smart choices that are convenient and that help us to lose weight and optimize our health is important, and we should be making consciously healthy choices for our bodies and our minds.

This can be done by following a dietary plan, tweaking it to suit our specific needs, meal-prepping and freezing our own foods, and ensuring we stay away from the snacks when we're shopping.

We need to have a plan when it comes to preparing our meals and when we're shopping for groceries so that we can avoid falling into old nutrition habits.

For many seniors, the slow march of poor nutrition happens when their kids grow up and they're left to their own devices. Suddenly, cooking for one or two is not particularly appealing, and when we throw mobility issues into the mix, this march can speed up to a run.

Here's the thing; we don't really need to stop cooking for a lot of people, we just need to know what to cook so that we can properly store and freeze the healthy, nutritious foods we need to be healthy and lose weight.

I'm sure you're eager for great, easy-to-follow recipes, a convenient 4-week meal plan, and a comprehensive shopping list to help you plan your meals, so let's get into the details and place the final piece of your health and fitness puzzle.

Chapter 6

4-WEEK MEAL PLAN WITH SHOPPING LIST

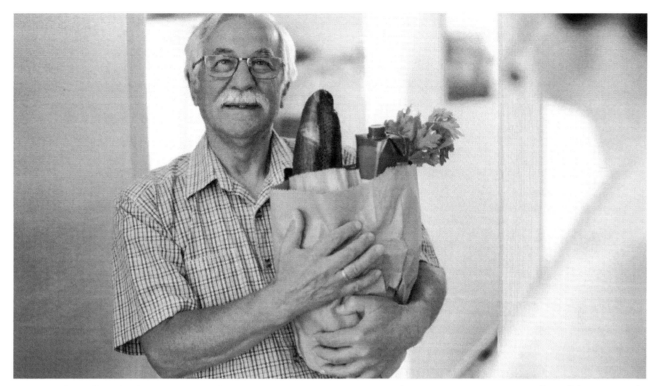

This final chapter is dedicated to some quick, convenient, yet healthy meals that you can prepare in advance and freeze or refrigerate for later. Each of these meals comes with a shopping list as well as a recipe.

Feel free to modify each of these to suit your specific dietary needs and tastes, but do be mindful of additional hidden calories in anything you add to your dish.

Icons Key

 = Time   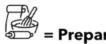 **= Serving size**   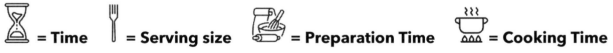 **= Preparation Time**   **= Cooking Time**

Breakfast Recipes

QUICK AND EASY SPINACH OMELET

 10 minutes   **1 person**   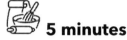 **5 minutes**   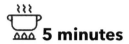 **5 minutes**

Nutritional Facts: 255 calories, 19g fat, 3g carbohydrates, 17g protein

Ingredients

1. Large eggs, 2
2. Extra-virgin olive oil, 1 tsp
3. Spinach, fresh or frozen, 1 cup
4. Cheddar cheese, shredded, 2 tbsp
5. Salt and pepper to taste

Directions

- Whisk your eggs in a small bowl.
- Heat a small, non-stick skillet over medium heat.
- Pour your oil into the pan and allow to heat up.
- Turn your head down to medium-low.
- Pour your whisked eggs into the skillet, immediately stirring with a spatula.
- Tilt your pan slightly to cover the edges of the pan with egg.
- Cover the skillet for about 3 minutes or until the egg is cooked on top.
- Switch the stove off and remove the skillet from the heat.
- If you're using frozen spinach, place it in a small bowl and microwave for 2 to 3 minutes or until properly defrosted and warm.
- Add the cheese and spinach to the omelet.
- Flip the corner of the omelet over and slide onto a plate.`
- Sprinkle with salt and pepper to taste.

SPINACH AND BLUEBERRY SMOOTHIE

 5 minutes   **1 person**   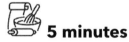 **5 minutes**   **N/A**

Nutritional Facts: 342 calories, 4g fat, 67g carbohydrates, 11g protein

Ingredients

1. Spinach, frozen or fresh, 1 cup.
2. Blueberries, frozen or fresh, 1 cup–feel free to swap out for any seasonal berry.
3. Rolled or fine oats, ¼ cup.
4. Honey or maple syrup, 2 tsps–optional for sweetness.

5. Oat or other plant-based milk, or half-fat cow's milk—1 ¼ cup.

Directions

- Place all of your ingredients in a blender or the supplied container for a hand blender.
- Blend on medium-low speed until all of the ingredients are combined and drinkable.
- Switch the blender off and decant the smoothie into a tall glass.

YOGURT PROTEIN BOWL

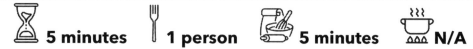 5 minutes 1 person 5 minutes N/A

Nutritional Facts: 337 calories, 7g fat, 33g carbohydrates, 32g protein

Ingredients

1. Yogurt plain, 1 cup.
2. Blueberries, frozen or fresh, ⅓ cup—feel free to swap out for any seasonal berry.
3. Walnuts, chopped, 3 tbsp.

Directions

- Decant your yogurt into a small bowl.
- Add your blueberries—feel free to thaw in some room temperature water if frozen.
- Mix blueberries in the yogurt.
- Sprinkle the walnuts over the top.

ROLLED OATS

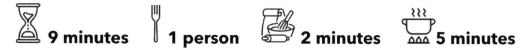 9 minutes 1 person 2 minutes 5 minutes

Nutritional Facts: 290 calories, 9g fat, 58g carbohydrates, 18g protein

Ingredients

1. Rolled or fine oats, 1 ½ cups.
2. Water, 2 cups.
3. Pinch of salt.
4. Plant-based or half-fat cow's milk, ¼ cup.

Directions

- Place your water and pinch of salt in a pot—if microwaving, place in a microwave-proof bowl.

- Put your oats in the water and allow to sit for 2 minutes.
- Switch your stove on to medium heat—alternatively set your microwave to high and cook for 2 minutes.
- Stove-top oats can be covered and boiled for 2 minutes, stirring occasionally.
- Switch the stove off.
- Remove the pot from the heat.
- Allow both microwaved and stove-top oats to rest for 2 minutes.
- Carefully decant the oats into a serving bowl.
- Add the milk and stir.

Lunch Recipes

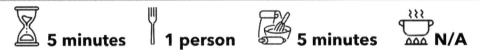

WHITE BEAN SALAD

5 minutes 1 person 5 minutes N/A

Nutritional Facts: 362 calories, 15g fat, 40g carbohydrates, 14g protein

Ingredients

1. Kale and broccoli slaw mix, 1 bag, 10 ounces—feel free to swap for other seasonal salad mix.
2. Cannellini beans, canned, no salt added, 15 ounces.
3. Plain yogurt, ¼ cup.
4. Salt and pepper to taste.

Directions

- Wash your salad mix and decant onto a plate or salad bowl.
- Open your can of cannellini beans and strain.
- Wash the cannellini beans and strain thoroughly once more.
- In a separate small bowl, mix plain yogurt with salt and pepper, and fresh lemon juice if you like.
- Place the cannellini beans on the salad greens.
- Drizzle plain yogurt over the top and toss.

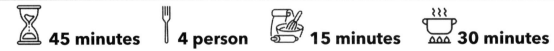

SATAY CHICKEN SALAD

45 minutes 4 person 15 minutes 30 minutes

Nutritional Facts: 393 calories, 15g fat, 32g carbohydrates, 30g protein

Ingredients

1. Sweet potatoes, scrubbed and cut into 1-inch cubes, 1 pound.

2. Olive Oil, 1 ½ tsps.
3. Salt and pepper to taste.
4. Peanut butter, 1 tbsp.
5. Honey, ½ tbsp.
6. Salad mix, 1 bag, 10 ounces.
7. Chicken breast, precooked and shredded, 2 cups.
8. Peanuts, chopped and salted, ¼ cup.

Directions

- Preheat your oven to 425 degrees Fahrenheit.
- Line a baking sheet with foil.
- Toss sweet potatoes in olive oil.
- Arrange sweet potato cubes on baking sheet.
- Place in the oven and roast for about 20 minutes.
- Switch the oven off.
- Remove the sweet potatoes and place them to one side to cool.
- In a small mixing bowl, mix peanut butter, honey, and olive oil—satay dressing
- Divide salad mix between bowls.
- Top each bowl of salad mix with 1 ½ cups chicken.
- Add ½ cup roast sweet potatoes to the bowl.
- Drizzle the satay dressing over the top of the and toss lightly.
- Sprinkle a few chopped peanuts over the top of the salad and serve.

CHICKEN AND SPINACH SOUP

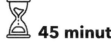 **45 minutes**   **6 person** 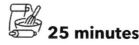 **25 minutes** 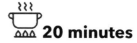 **20 minutes**

Nutritional Facts: 271 calories, 5g fat, 30g carbohydrates, 26g protein

Ingredients

1. Olive oil, 1 tbsp
2. Onion, 1 ½ cups
3. Garlic, fresh or dried, 1 tbsp
4. Cannellini beans, canned, no salt added, 15 ounces.
5. Chicken breast, precooked and shredded, 2 cups.
6. Potatoes, peeled and diced, 2 medium.
7. Water, 6 cups.
8. Salt and pepper, to taste.
9. Thyme, dried or fresh, 1 tsp
10. Spinach, fresh or frozen, 3 cups.
11. Lemon juice, fresh or store-bought, 2 tbsp.

Directions

- Place a large pot on the stove over medium heat.
- Heat the olive oil.
- Add the onions, stirring occasionally.
- Cook the onions until soft, about 5 minutes.
- Add the garlic.
- Cook the garlic, stirring constantly, until soft and fragrant, about 1 minute.
- Add the beans, potatoes, chicken, water, and salt and pepper to taste.
- Stir to mix.
- Turn the stove down to low heat.
- Cover the pot and simmer until potatoes are tender, about 25 minutes.
- Add the spinach to the pot.
- Turn up the heat to medium and bring to the boil for about 2 minutes.
- Turn off the stove and remove from the heat.
- Add the lemon juice and stir.
- Plate and enjoy.

Cooled soup can be portioned and frozen for reheating to enjoy at lunch or as a light supper.

RUSSIAN DRESSING FILLER

The recipe below is a sandwich and wrap filler or can be added to a bowl of greens. It freezes well and can be made in bulk.

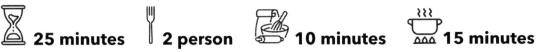 **25 minutes**   **2 person**   **10 minutes**   **15 minutes**

Nutritional Facts: 343 calories, 12g fat, 44g carbohydrates, 16g protein

Ingredients

For the Russian Dressing

1. Mayonnaise, 2 tbsps.
2. Ketchup, 2 tbsps.
3. Onion, diced, 1 tsp.
4. Pickle or other relish, diced, 1 tsp.

For the Filling

5. Mushrooms, sliced, 1 cup—omit or replace if not wanted.
6. Onion, diced, 2 tbsps.
7. Olive oil, 1 tbsp.
8. Spinach, frozen or fresh, 1 cup.
9. Salt and pepper to taste.

10. Deli meat, your choice, or shredded chicken, 2 slices or ½ cup shredded chicken.
11. Cheddar cheese, shredded, ¼ cup.
12. Wraps, whole grain bread, or salad mix—depending on your serving method.

Directions

For the Russian Dressing

- In a small bowl, whisk the mayonnaise and ketchup until combined well and smooth.
- Add the diced pickles/relish, and onions, and stir until combined.

For the Filling

- Switch the stove on to medium heat.
- Place olive oil in a medium-sized non-stick skillet.
- Add the onions and mushrooms to the skilled—omit the mushrooms if not desired.
- Stir onions and mushrooms until soft, about 4 minutes.
- Add the spinach and cook, stirring occasionally until the spinach is withered, between 2 and 5 minutes.
- Add your salt and pepper to taste.
- Switch the stove off and remove the skillet from the stove.
- Once cooled, drizzle your dressing over the mixture and stir generously.
- Halve your portion, freezing or refrigerating one half, and serve the other on whole grain bread, a wrap, or over salad greens.
- Add your favorite deli meat or shredded chicken and your cheese when serving.

Supper Recipes

All of the supper and lunch meals can be swapped so that you can eat your higher calorie, heavier meal at lunch, enjoying a light meal at supper.

PARSLEY AND WALNUT PESTO PASTA

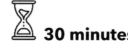 **30 minutes**   **4-2 cups per person**   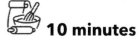 **10 minutes**   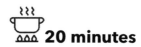 **20 minutes**

Nutritional Facts: 514 calories, 27g fat, 43g carbohydrates, 31g protein—per serving

The sauce for this recipe can be separated and frozen for later meals.

Ingredients

For the Sauce

1. Walnuts, chopped, ¾ cup.
2. Parsley leaves, fresh, 1 cup.
3. Garlic, peeled and crushed, 2 cloves, or 1 tsp dried.
4. Salt to taste, about ⅛ tsp.
5. Pepper to taste.
6. Olive oil, 3 tbsp.
7. Chicken breast, precooked, shredded, 1 ½ cups.
8. Peppers, any color, chopped, ½ cup,

For the Pasta

9. Penne or fusilli pasta, whole-wheat, 1 ¾ cups.
10. Water, 2 ½ cups.
11. Salt, a pinch.

Directions

For the Sauce

- Place your parsley, garlic, olive oil, walnuts, salt and pepper in a blender.
- Pulse on high until the walnuts are ground and the consistency resembles pesto.
- Heat your stove to medium.
- Pour your sauce into a medium-sized skillet and bring to a simmer—about 3 minutes.
- Turn the heat down to low.
- Add your shredded chicken and peppers and allow to cook on low heat for about another 5 minutes.
- Turn the stove off and remove the skillet from the stove.

For the Pasta

- Pour your water into a medium to large pot.
- Add a pinch of salt.
- Switch the stove on to medium-high heat.
- Allow the water to come to a boil.
- Turn the heat down to medium.
- Add the pasta and cook, stirring occasionally, about 10 minutes.
- Turn off the stove.
- Carefully scoop about ½ cup pasta water to your pesto mix.
- Mix the water with the pesto until combined well.
- Strain your pasta.
- Serve 2 cups of cooked pasta with a quarter of your pesto.

- Toss the pasta until well coated with the pesto.
- You can top your pasta with parmesan or a light drizzle of shredded cheddar cheese if you like.
- The remaining pesto and chicken sauce can be cooled and frozen for future meals.

BROCCOLI CHICKEN STIR FRY

The chicken can be swapped out in this recipe for boneless fish, tofu, or beef strips.

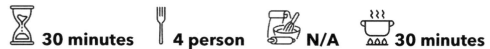 **30 minutes**   **4 person**   **N/A**   **30 minutes**

Nutritional Facts: 341 calories, 20g fat, 12g carbohydrates, 29g protein—per serving

Ingredients

1. Lemon juice, fresh or store-bought, 2 tbsps.
2. Ginger, dry or fresh, 1 tbsp.
3. Garlic, minced or dried, 3 tsps.
4. Soy sauce, low sodium, 1 tbsp.
5. Olive oil, 1 tbsp
6. Onions, diced, 2 tbsp.
7. Sugar, 1 tsp.
8. Water, ¼ cup.
9. Chicken, strips, 3 cups—fish, seafood, or tender beef flank can substitute.
10. Broccoli florets, frozen or fresh, 4 cups.
11. Peppers, in any color, sliced into strips, 3 cups.

Directions

- In a small pot, combine the lemon juice, soya sauce, sugar, oil, ginger, garlic, and half your water.
- Place the pot on the stove and heat at medium to low.
- Allow to simmer, stirring occasionally until the sugar is melted and the sauce is hot, between 7 and 10 minutes.
- Remove from the heat.
- Place a large skillet on the stove, do not turn the heat down.
- Dry fry your onions until they are soft but not browned.
- Add the chicken or preferred meat or tofu and brown for about 5 minutes.
- Put the remainder of your ingredients in your skillet.
- Once the liquid begins boiling, add your sauce.

- Turn the stove to low, tossing your ingredients occasionally to ensure even cooking, about 10 minutes.
- Finally, turn your stove up to medium-high heat and cook for a further 5 minutes, stirring continuously until the stirfry is a golden brown color.
- Switch the stove off and serve hot.

This recipe can be cooled and frozen for reheating.

PESTO STUFFED PEPPERS

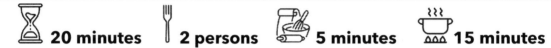

⏳ **20 minutes** 🍴 **2 persons** 🥣 **5 minutes** 🍲 **15 minutes**

Nutritional Facts: 347 calories, 19g fat, 41g carbohydrates, 26g protein—per serving

Ingredients

1. Chicken pesto sauce from Parsley and Walnut, defrosted, 2 servings.
2. Olive oil, 2 tbsps
3. Bell pepper, your preferred color, halved and seeded.
4. Cheddar, shredded, ½ cup.

Directions

Preheat your oven to 375 degrees Fahrenheit.

- Line a baking sheet with foil.
- Lightly coat each of your pepper halves with olive oil.
- Scoop 1 serving of your parsley, pesto, and chicken sauce into each pepper half.
- Place the peppers on your baking sheet, making sure they are balanced.
- Place in the oven and bake for about 15 minutes or until the pepper is soft to the touch and the sauce is bubbling.
- Switch the oven off.
- Carefully remove the baking sheet from the oven and place to one side.
- Sprinkle half of your cheddar on one pepper and the other half on the other pepper.
- Serve hot.

STUFFED SWEET POTATOES

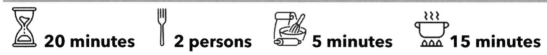

⏳ **20 minutes** 🍴 **2 persons** 🥣 **5 minutes** 🍲 **15 minutes**

Nutritional Facts: 472 calories, 7g fat, 85g carbohydrates, 21g protein—per serving

Ingredients

1. Sweet potato, scrubbed, 1 large.
2. Russian dressing filler, defrosted, 2 portions.
3. Chicken, shredded, 1 cup—can be replaced with ½ cup diced deli meat.
4. Cheddar cheese, shredded, ½ cup.
5. Parsley for dressing, if desired.

Directions

- Prick your sweet potato with a fork as deep and as generously as possible.
- Place sweet potato in the microwave and cook on high for about 10 minutes or until a skewer pierces through.
- Carefully remove the sweet potato from the microwave—both the potato and dish will be hot.
- Using an oven mitt, halve your sweet potato.
- Scoop about half the middle of your potato halved out into a medium-sized bowl.
- Combine your Russian dressing mixture and shredded chicken or deli meat to your bowl.
- Mix the potato and dressing until well combined.
- Return mixture to the microwave for 1 to 2 minutes to heat evenly.
- Plate the potato half and scoop your mixture into the potato.
- Top with shredded cheese.
- The other half can be frozen and reheated for another meal.

Snacks

- ¼ cup dry-roasted unsalted almonds—206 calories
- 1 medium orange—62 calories
- 1 large pear—131 calories
- 10 dried walnut—131 calories
- ½ cup raspberries—32 calories

SHOPPING LIST

Meat	Vegetables	Fruits	Dairy	Other	Checkbox
	Spinach–fresh or frozen				☐
	Salad mix– brocolli, kale, lettuce				☐
	Sweet potato				☐
	Potatoes				☐
	Garlic				☐
	Thyme				☐
	Onions				☐
	Parsley				☐
	Ginger				☐
	Brocolli– fresh or frozen				☐
		Blueberries or other seasonal berries– fresh			☐

		Oranges		☐
		Pears		☐
		Raspberries or other season berry–fresh		☐
			Cheddar cheese-shredded	☐
			Plant–based or half–fat milk	☐
			Cannellini Beans	☐
				Eggs ☐
				Olive Oil ☐
				Salt ☐
				Pepper ☐
				Rolled or fine oats ☐
				Honey or maple syrup ☐

				Peanut butter	☐
				Peanuts	☐
				Wraps	☐
				Whole-grain bread	☐
				Mayonnaise	☐
				Ketchup	☐
				Soy sauce- low sodium	☐
				Walnuts	☐
				Almonds	☐
Chicken breasts					☐
Chicken strips or preferred protein					☐

WEEKLY MEAL PLAN

Monday	Tuesday	Wednesday	Thursday
Breakfast: Quick and Easy Spinach Omelet	**Breakfast:** Spinach and Blueberry Smoothie	**Breakfast:** Rolled Oats	**Breakfast:** Yogurt Protein Bowl
Lunch: Satay Chicken Salad	**Lunch:** Russian Dressing Filler Wrap or Sandwich	**Lunch:** White Bean Salad	**Lunch:** Chicken and Spinach Soup
Supper: Brocolli Chicken Stirfry	**Supper:** Pesto Stuffed Peppers	**Supper:** Parsley and Walnut Pesto Pasta	**Supper:** Pesto Stuffed Peppers
Snack: 1 pear and 1/2 cup raspberries	**Snack:** walnuts and 1 large orange	**Snack:** Unsalted almonds and 1 pear	**Snack:** 1 large orange and 1/2 cup raspberries

Friday	Saturday	Sunday	Calorie Notes
Breakfast: Quick and Easy Spinach Omelet	**Breakfast:** Spinach and Blueberry Smoothie	**Breakfast:** Rolled Oats	
Lunch: Satay Chicken Salad	**Lunch:** Russian Dressing Filler Wrap or Sandwich	**Lunch:** White Bean Salad	
Supper: Brocolli Chicken Stirfry	**Supper:** Pesto Stuffed Peppers	**Supper:** Parsley and Walnut Pesto Pasta	
Snack: 1 pear and 1/2 cup raspberries	**Snack:** walnuts and 1 large orange	**Snack:** Unsalted almonds and 1 pear	

CONCLUSION

Our health as we age is so much more than taking medication and keeping up with doctor's appointments and we can sometimes feel that everything from a changing appetite to mobility limitations, and our new lifestyle is working against us when it comes to our strength and our health.

The reality is that we don't have to be a victim to the ticking clock of time and we do play a very large role in maintaining our health, building a strong body, and living a life that embraces independence, mobility, and flexibility as well as supporting our bodies nutrition needs.

Throughout the course of this book, you've been supplied with all the tools you need to build the body and the life you want. Now is the time to set your health and wellness goals, change your mindset and lose the weight you need for a strong, happy body.

Remember, getting older isn't something we should fear. Instead, it's a time to begin a new chapter in our lives where we can choose the life we want to live.

Today is the beginning of *Your 4-Week Journey to Renew Your Body Image* with your new 5-minute yoga plan.

Without your voice we don't exist.
Please, support us and leave a honest review on Amazon

Just scan this QR code with your phone's camera and leave a review

Printed in Great Britain
by Amazon

0989ade7-820b-407a-be90-1ac848972708R02